THE BEGINNER'S GUIDE TO COSMETIC BREAST SURGERY

A FULLY ILLUSTRATED, IN DEPTH GUIDE TO ALL ELEMENTS OF COSMETIC BREAST SURGERY

ANNABELLE BAUGH, FOUNDER OF COSMETIC SURGERY ADVANCEMENTS

MR DOUGLAS MCGEORGE, FRCS (PLAST)

CONTENTS

INTRODUCTION

Who is This Book For?	3
A Message from Annabelle	5
Cosmetic Surgery Advancements (CSA) Consultant Register	8
Unlocking the Secrets of this Book: A Comprehensive Guide	11

1. THE FOUNDATIONS

Introduction	15
Regulatory Medical Bodies	17
1. UK and Ireland	18
2. US and Canada	21
3. Australia and New Zealand	25
Worldwide Plastic Surgery Organisations	27
How to Find a Plastic Surgeon	30
Ten Questions to Ask Your Plastic Surgeon	32

2. THE FUNDAMENTALS

A. Surgical and Anaesthesia Risks and Complications	37
B. Breast Augmentation Surgery	43
1. Breast Augmentation With Implants	44
2. Autologous Breast Fat Transfer	67
3. Breast Implant Illness (BII), Breast Implant Associated Large Cell Lymphoma (BIA-ALCL) and Breast Implant Associated Squamous Cell Carcinoma (BIA-SCC)	76
4. Monitoring Breast Implants for Rupture	84
5. Breast Implant Revision, Removal or Implant Replacement Surgery	90
6. Extra Large Breast Implants	98
7. Breast Implant Manufacturers	107

C. Breast Uplift and Reduction Surgery	113
1. Breast Uplift With or Without Implants	114
2. Breast Reduction Surgery	125
D. Cosmetic Nipple Surgery	134
1. Areola Reduction Surgery	135
2. Inverted Nipple Correction	139
E. Breast Surgery Scar Treatments	142

3. TRAVELLING ABROAD FOR COSMETIC SURGERY

Travelling Abroad for Cosmetic Surgery	151

4. ADVICE AND GUIDANCE

Advice and Guidance	159

5. FINAL THOUGHTS FROM ANNABELLE

1. Final Thoughts From Annabelle	165
Research and Resources	167

INTRODUCTION

WHO IS THIS BOOK FOR?

Let me make some challenging assumptions about you before I do anything else

TO MAKE sure I endeavoured to meet what you're looking for and provide you with the information you need to make informed and educated decisions, I had to put together a few guesses about you in order to write this book.

- You're thinking about having cosmetic or plastic breast surgery, but you don't know where to look for an appropriately qualified physician.
- You want to be sure your friend or family member receiving cosmetic or plastic breast surgery is in good hands and has an understanding of the procedure they are considering.
- You've undergone cosmetic or plastic breast surgery and are disappointed with the results and you want to make sure your revision surgery is successful.

. . .

JUST A LITTLE WORD about mental health

You can embrace your individuality and the life you want to lead by having cosmetic or plastic surgery. However, it is not a "cure all". Working with a trained therapist rather than a plastic surgeon is the best place to start if you are having problems with your relationships, or mental health.

"Reclaim an incredible sense of self"

A MESSAGE FROM ANNABELLE

Are you considering cosmetic surgery or just curious? Either way, it is important to have reliable information to make informed decisions. Cosmetic surgery is a rapidly growing industry, and unfortunately, some physicians and clinics prioritise profits over patient safety. This leaves patients in the hands of 'physicians' who have no plastic surgery qualifications or training.

This is why the cosmetic surgery industry and cosmetic surgery in general has become an extremely dangerous place for vulnerable patients. With numerous cases reported of horrific complications, permanent disfigurement, and even death when cosmetic surgery is performed by physicians who are not qualified plastic surgeons.

As someone who has had various cosmetic surgery procedures, including three breast augmentations, I know first hand the desire to alter your appearance. The alarming promotion of cosmetic surgeons who have very little, if any training in plastic surgery, has led me to want to raise awareness of the potential dangers, and want to encourage a more thoughtful and critical approach to choosing a surgeon.

While there is a lot of information available online, I wanted to provide the information in a format that is easy to read and understand. I have also included the key questions to ask your surgeon about your chosen breast cosmetic or plastic surgery procedure(s) to ensure you can make informed decisions. By shedding light on the lack of regulation around cosmetic surgery, I hope to empower you to make better informed choices, and find a qualified plastic surgeon, who will put your health above all else.

About my Co Author Mr Douglas McGeorge FRCS Plast

Sections of "The Beginner's Guide to Cosmetic Surgery and Staying Safe" have been prepared in collaboration with Mr Douglas Mcgeorge, a well known UK plastic surgeon; who has been on the specialist GMC register since the 26th August 1981. Sections that have been checked by Douglas will be marked by a notation that they have been medically reviewed by Douglas Mcgeorge.

Douglas McGeorge is dedicated to sharing his knowledge and supporting others and his achievements include:

- Past President of The British Association of Aesthetic Plastic Surgeons (BAAPS) and currently closely involved in the training and standards of cosmetic plastic surgery as a Council Member.
- Full member of the British Association of Plastic, Reconstructive Aesthetic Surgeons (BAPRAS)
- Full member of the International Society of Aesthetic Plastic Surgeons (ISAPS)
- Accredited Platinum BUPA Consultant Surgeon
- Contributor to the Prince's Trust over many years.
- Trustee of the Scar Free Foundation for some 14 years.
- Awarded an MBE for his charitable services.

. . .

PASSIONATE ABOUT EDUCATING people regarding the importance of choosing a qualified plastic surgeon, Douglas has been featured in the documentary series The Ugly Face of Beauty on channel 4. Additionally he has been featured in the New York Times, BBC News, The Guardian, Tatler, Spears, The Daily Mail and My Face My Body. Without doubt Douglas is widely considered one of the top recommended plastic surgeons in the UK. In addition to working as a plastic surgeon, Douglas has also published numerous research papers on a variety of topics.

Evidence-Based Research and Studies

Our compilation of references encompasses a blend of internal research and external sources, with a predominant inclusion of scientific publications that are accessible through external links. Our commitment is centred on delivering the latest, unbiased, factual, and evidence based information. This ensures that the content we provide empowers you to make well informed decisions based on reliable and up to date insights.

Whether you're a potential patient or simply curious about the industry, hopefully you will find this book is an invaluable resource.

"Take back control and live your best life"

COSMETIC SURGERY ADVANCEMENTS (CSA) CONSULTANT REGISTER

Are you looking for certified plastic surgeons you can trust? Look no further than the CSA Consultant Register! We connect you with qualified plastic surgeons who meet the highest standards in their field.

All our surgeons in the US are certified by the American Board of Plastic Surgery, while in Canada, they are certified by The Royal College of Physicians and Surgeons of Canada. Our plastic surgeons in the UK are consultant plastic surgeons on the GMC specialist register, which ensures not only their credibility but also their expertise.

So what makes us different? At CSA, we take extra measures to verify all CSA members and confirm their registration with the appropriate medical bodies, conducting annual checks to guarantee that they maintain their credibility year after year.

Your safety and satisfaction are our priorities. Discover the difference of choosing <u>CSA Consultant Register</u> for your plastic and cosmetic surgery needs.

My Motivation

I'm Annabelle, Founder of the Cosmetic Surgery Advancements (CSA) website and consultant directory. CSA began when I discovered that my Allergan implants had been withdrawn due to a link with a rare lymphatic cancer, known as 'Breast Implant Associated Anaplastic Large Cell Lymphoma (BIA-ALCL). After finding various websites with different information I decided to collate it and put it into a blog, to provide a trustworthy resource for other women facing similar concerns.

After being approached by numerous women who were unsure how to find a plastic surgeon, I realised that a reputable directory of verified plastic surgeons would be the best way I could support anyone who was considering cosmetic or plastic surgery.

Choosing the Right Plastic Surgeon is ESSENTIAL for Your Safety

I initially chose my UK plastic surgeon based on a friend's recommendation, and luckily, Douglas was a properly qualified plastic surgeon on the GMC Specialist register. Over 20 years later, I'm still happy with the results of my plastic surgery. But I also recognise that things could have turned out differently if I hadn't been under the care of a qualified, compassionate plastic surgeon.

The Importance of Stricter Regulation in Cosmetic Surgery

Unfortunately, regulatory authorities and lawmakers around the world are currently failing patients who are seeking cosmetic surgery, due to lack of regulation. Subsequently allowing many cosmetic surgery websites and directories to profit by promoting medical practitioners, non-specialist surgeons, or those without appropriate surgical training, who are performing cosmetic surgery. This is putting patients at risk for life-changing complications or even death.

That's why I created the <u>CSA Consultant Directory</u>, to protect patients from unscrupulous 'cosmetic surgeons.'

Choose Wisely and Stay True to Yourself

Who you choose to perform your cosmetic surgery is a personal decision. Just make sure they are a properly qualified plastic surgeon and don't rely on testimonials or star ratings on websites. Your cosmetic surgery journey should be about feeling comfortable in your body and embracing self love.

UNLOCKING THE SECRETS OF THIS BOOK: A COMPREHENSIVE GUIDE

- **The Foundations** are covered in the first section. There are numerous medical organisations and bodies you should be aware of, along with information about how to verify a surgeon's training and experience.
- **The Fundamentals** of the most popular cosmetic and plastic breast surgery procedures are covered in the second section, and key questions to ask your plastic surgeon. This information is to assist you in making decisions that will not only provide you with the best results, but also benefit you in the long run.
- **Travelling Abroad** and all the factors to take into account before travelling abroad for breast cosmetic or plastic surgery are covered in the third part.
- **Advice** on how to make final decisions and discuss them with friends and family can be found in this section.

"You have the power to determine your own boundaries"

1. THE FOUNDATIONS

INTRODUCTION

Feeling overwhelmed by the various types of practitioners and facilities that can perform cosmetic surgery procedures? Don't worry - you are not alone. In this section, I'll provide you with an overview of the different types of practitioners and facilities that can provide cosmetic surgery procedures, as well as the regulations and regulatory bodies involved.

It's important to note that the lack of regulation around cosmetic surgery is a global problem. While some procedures may seem relatively simple to perform, the potential complications when any cosmetic surgery procedure is performed incorrectly, can be extremely serious.

But with the aid of this information, you will be equipped with the knowledge required to select the ideal plastic surgeon and facility for your cosmetic surgery requirements. The material that follows will help you verify the credentials and licensing of surgeons and facilities practising cosmetic and plastic surgery procedures, in order to safeguard yourself and the standard of care you receive.

So, whether you are considering cosmetic surgery or just

interested in learning more about it, this section is a great place to start.

"Nothing beats living with confidence"

REGULATORY MEDICAL BODIES

Around the world, there are numerous medical regulatory and professional bodies that play a vital role in maintaining high standards of care and ensuring patient safety. Unfortunately, the cosmetic surgery industry has seen a steady rise in unqualified practitioners providing cosmetic surgery. Consequently it is essential to check your cosmetic surgeons' qualifications before proceeding. This section covers the regulatory medical bodies in the:

- UK and Ireland
- US and Canada
- Australia and New Zealand.

1. UK AND IRELAND

Licensed Facilities

Care Quality Commission (CQC)
In the UK, the CQC, or Care Quality Commission, is a public body responsible for regulating and inspecting facilities that provide cosmetic surgery. They are part of the Department of Health and Social Care and inspect healthcare facilities in England to ensure that they provide safe, effective, compassionate, and high-quality care.

If a facility has been registered with the CQC, individuals can expect certain standards. For example, they must receive care or treatment that is tailored to their needs and preferences and patients must be treated with dignity and respect at all times. The equipment must be clean and suitable, and staff should only provide care and treatment appropriate to their role. In the event that something goes wrong with your care and treatment, the provider of your care must tell you what has happened and provide support to rectify any ongoing issues relating to the error.

You can check CQC inspection reports and ratings for a

cosmetic surgery facility, on the care provider's pages on the CQC website.

[CQC Provider Search]()

Verifying the Accreditation of Plastic Surgeons

The General Medical Council

When it comes to cosmetic surgery, it's essential to be well-informed about the procedures and the professionals who will be performing them. The General Medical Council (GMC) plays a significant role in ensuring the safety and quality of cosmetic surgery in the UK. Their guidelines for cosmetic surgery help maintain a high standard of care and protect patients from potential risks. However, in the UK whilst all individuals carrying out surgical procedures must be GMC registered, not all surgeons carrying out cosmetic procedures are on Specialist Registers. The British Association of Aesthetic Plastic Surgeons is pushing to make this mandatory.

Professional Standards and Qualifications

In order to practise as a plastic surgeon in the UK, a surgeon must first be registered with the GMC and hold a licence to practise. Additionally, the GMC Specialist Register is a list of doctors and surgeons who are eligible for appointment in consultant posts in the NHS, which is a pretty big deal!

Plastic surgeons registered with the General Medical Council (GMC) Specialist Register of plastic surgery will have the letters FRCS (PLAST) after their name. This means that they have been formally trained and UK qualified in plastic surgery

[GMC Specialist Register]()

Plastic Surgery Organizations

British Association of Aesthetic Plastic Surgeons (BAAPS)

The British Association of Aesthetic Plastic Surgeons (BAAPS) is a professional non profit organisation dedicated to promoting safety, innovation, and ethical practice in aesthetic plastic surgery. Members must be registered on the Specialist Register of Plastic Surgery of the General Medical Council, undergo regular audits, and attend educational conferences to maintain their membership. By choosing a BAAPS member surgeon, you can feel confident that they have met the highest standards of training and expertise within the field of cosmetic surgery.

BAAPS Member Search

British Association of Plastic, Reconstructive and Aesthetic Surgeons (BAPRAS)

The British Association of Plastic, Reconstructive, and Aesthetic Surgeons (BAPRAS) is a non profit organisation consisting of highly skilled plastic surgeons who specialise in plastic, reconstructive, and aesthetic surgery. BAPRAS strives to promote innovation in teaching, learning, and research within the field. The organisation is governed by elected officers and council members who are also trustees of the association.

The members of BAPRAS are registered on the Specialist Register of Plastic Surgery of the General Medical Council dedicated to improving the lives of their patients and are passionate about their work. So, if you're looking for a plastic surgeon a BAPRAS member is a good indication of their surgical abilities.

BAPRAS Member Search

2. US AND CANADA

Licensed Facilities

In the United States and Canada, cosmetic surgery can be performed in a variety of healthcare facilities, including hospitals, ambulatory surgery centres, and private clinics. The licensing requirements for these facilities vary state by state and can be overseen by different licensing bodies. That is why if you are thinking about having surgery, it's crucial to confirm that the hospital where the procedure will be performed has a licence from one of the below organisations, which have rigorous regulations and routinely inspect facilities to make sure they are up to the set standards:

- The American Association for Accreditation of Ambulatory Surgery Facilities - **AAAASF**
- The Accreditation Association for Ambulatory Health Care - **AAAHC**
- **The Joint Commission**

. . .

It's important to note that licensing requirements can vary by state and that not all states require licensing or accreditation for cosmetic surgery facilities. Before undergoing any cosmetic procedure, it's important to check the licensing body for the facility where your procedure will take place.

Verifying the Accreditation of Plastic Surgeons

In America and Canada any physician with a medical licence can perform cosmetic surgery, regardless of their training or experience.

The American Board of Medical Specialties - ABMS

Visit the Federation of State Medical Boards (FSMB) for an online directory and to contact your specific state medical board for information regarding their state medical licence, including "active, unrestricted" licence status verification and the procedure for formal patient complaints.

FSMB Online Directory

The American Board of Plastic Surgeons - ABPS

The American Board of Plastic Surgery - ABPS is a non-profit organisation that is responsible for certifying plastic surgeons in the United States. The purpose of the ABPS is to ensure that patients receive safe and effective care from qualified plastic surgeons who have met rigorous educational and training requirements.

To become board certified by the ABPS, a surgeon must complete a comprehensive training program in plastic surgery, pass a rigorous written exam, and demonstrate their skills and knowledge in a clinical exam. Once certified, plastic surgeons must maintain their certification by participating in ongoing education and training to stay up-to-date with the latest advances in their field. By providing certification for plastic surgeons, the ABPS helps to ensure that patients receive high-quality care from qualified providers.

The ABPS website has a search function that allows you to verify whether a surgeon is board certified by the ABPS. You can search for a surgeon by name, state, or specialty on the ABPS website to see if they are certified by the board. An alert to "See FSMB" will show in the certification status column if the ABPS receives notice of a state medical board action. By clicking the link, more details are available from the Federation of State Medical Boards (FSMB).

ABPS Member Search

Royal College of Physicians and Surgeons of Canada (RCPSC)

The Royal College of Physicians and Surgeons of Canada (RCPSC) is a non-profit organisation that oversees the national standards for medical education and continuing professional development of all surgeons including plastic surgeons in Canada. The ABMS recommends verifying the certification of a physician with a Canadian specialties plastic surgery certification using the member search function.

RCPSC Member Search

Plastic Surgery Organizations

American Society of Plastic Surgeons (ASPS)

The American Society of Plastic Surgeons (ASPS) is the largest plastic surgery specialty non profit organisation in the world. To be a member of the ASPS plastic surgeons need to be certified by the American Board of Plastic Surgery (ABPS) or by the Royal College of Physicians and Surgeons of Canada. ASPS represents 92% of all board-certified plastic surgeons in the United States and more than 11,000 plastic surgeons worldwide. When you choose a doctor who is a member of ASPS, you can rest assured that your surgeon is a qualified Board Registered Plastic Surgeon. You can check if your plastic surgeon is a member by using the search function on the website.

The Canadian Society of Plastic Surgeons (CSPS)

The Canadian Society of Plastic Surgeons (CSPS) is a non profit organisation and is composed of qualified plastic surgeons in Canada. CSPS members are medical doctors who have chosen to specialise in plastic surgery and are well-trained in their field to obtain the best results for their patients. To check if a surgeon is a member of the CSPS simply use the search option on the website.

CSPS Member Search

3. AUSTRALIA AND NEW ZEALAND

Licensed Facilities

Verifying the Accreditation of Plastic Surgeons

Royal Australasian College of Physicians (RACS)

In Australia and New Zealand fellows of the RACS must be Specialist Plastic Surgeons, accredited by the Commonwealth Government of Australia, through the Australian Medical Council. The simplest way to check if a surgeon in Australia or New Zealand is a specialist plastic surgeon is to use the RACS search.

THE RACS CODE of conduct includes:

- Providing clinical care consistent with the prevailing standards of their specialty.

- Ensure that they remain competent and provide clinical care that is informed by current and relevant evidence.
- Manage only those patients whose clinical conditions are within the surgeon's scope of practice, giving consideration to individual training, experience, credentialing and current practice profile Participate in the emergency management of a patient when requested, when they are reasonably able to do so, and when refusal might adversely affect the outcome for the patient.
- Refer a patient to another clinician when the best procedure for the patient is not within their scope of practice.
- Be receptive to their patient seeking a second opinion, and assist the patient to obtain a second opinion if requested.
- Ensure elective and scheduled urgent procedures are performed in an institution capable of providing the appropriate level of perioperative care.

[RACS Member Search](#)

WORLDWIDE PLASTIC SURGERY ORGANISATIONS

Licensed Facilities

There is not a set of standards which are substantially approved for facilities where surgery is conducted, and in many countries, there are no laws governing cosmetic surgery.

Therefore if you are considering surgery it is important to check the facility where the procedure will be performed is licensed by one of the below organisations that have strict regulations and check facilities on a routine basis, to ensure they are meeting the required standards:

Joint Commission International (JCI)

The JCI works to improve patient safety and quality of health care in the international community and JCI-accredited facilities exist in more than 100 countries.

JCI Facilities Search

Verifying the Accreditation of Plastic Surgeons

It can be quite challenging to determine whether your plastic surgeon has had the necessary training, and in certain nations, being board-certified is not as rigorous a procedure as in others. Please be aware that the UK does not grant board accreditation, instead imposing incredibly rigorous standards on plastic surgeons to be listed on the specialty GMC register.

Determining the amount of experience your surgeon has can be very complicated because there isn't a universally accepted set of academic requirements to become a surgeon or perform cosmetic surgery procedures. This is why I advise to ensure the competence of your chosen plastic surgeon is a member of either the European Association of Plastic Surgeons (EURAPS) or the International Society of Aesthetic Plastic Surgery (ISAPS) if you are travelling outside of the UK, US, Canada, Australia, or New Zealand. These affiliations can serve as indicators of a surgeon's commitment to their field and their adherence to international standards.

European Association of Plastic Surgeons (EURAPS)

Countries in Europe have various regulations around the type of physician that can perform cosmetic surgery. The easiest way to know if you are in the hands of a fully qualified plastic surgeon is to check if they are a member of EURAPS by using the search facility provided on the website.

In order to be a member of EURAPS plastic surgeons need to be:

- Full members of the National Society of Plastic Surgeons (evidence of membership must be submitted)

- Fully qualified as Plastic Surgeons for a minimum period of three years (evidence of the date of the Board must be submitted)

EURAPS Member Search

International Society of Aesthetic Plastic Surgery (ISAPS)

Worldwide regulations differ in so many ways. If you are considering plastic surgery in another country, ISAPS membership is the simplest way to check if a surgeon is a fully qualified plastic surgeon.

- To apply for membership with ISAPS plastic surgeons need to:
- Maintain active membership in the national society of plastic surgery in the country where they practise.
- Be sponsored by two active or life ISAPS members.
- Provide a seven-year practice history beyond graduation from medical school.

ISAPS Member Search

"It's time to wake up the best version of YOU!"

HOW TO FIND A PLASTIC SURGEON

Finding a qualified and experienced plastic surgeon is a crucial step in achieving a safe and successful procedure, with the results you desire. With so many physicians performing cosmetic surgery, it can be overwhelming to decide who to trust.

Below is a list of essential factors to consider when selecting a plastic surgeon for your cosmetic or plastic surgery.

- *Experience:* Look for a surgeon who has vast experience in the procedure(s) you are considering. Ask:
  - Where they trained
  - How often do they perform the procedure in a month
  - How many times they have performed the procedure in the past three months
  - How many revision procedures they have performed due to complications in the past 12 months
- *Certification:* Ensure that the surgeon is registered with the appropriate medical body
- *Before and after photos:* Check the surgeon's portfolio for photos of previous patients' results - but remember you are only ever going to see a small selection of the very best of their work.

NB Not all plastic surgeons will have before and after patient photos. Some prefer not to provide patient photos as they feel they can be misleading and may create unrealistic expectations. After all cosmetic surgery isn't like choosing a hairstyle, your physiology and how you heal, as well as if there are any complications will impact the end result, so use caution when viewing patient photos.

• *Communication:* Choose a surgeon who is easy to communicate with, takes time to answer all your questions, and provides a way to contact them if you have follow up queries.

It's all about finding someone you trust and feel comfortable with. By doing thorough research, asking the right questions, and trusting your instincts, you can confidently select the best surgeon for your cosmetic or plastic surgery procedure.

"Feeling your best is empowering"

TEN QUESTIONS TO ASK YOUR PLASTIC SURGEON

1. How many times a month do you carry out this procedure?

Many cosmetic surgeons are capable of performing a variety of procedures, some of which are performed more frequently than others. You can find out if they have a lot of expertise with the procedure you are considering by asking this question.

2. What outcomes might I anticipate, and how long could they possibly last?

The evaluation from your plastic surgeon will establish whether you are a good candidate for the procedure and the long-term outcomes you can expect.

3. Which anaesthetic do you suggest using for this procedure? Your surgeon can recommend using one of a few different types of anaesthetic.

This will frequently involve IV sedation, local and general anaesthesia. If a general anaesthesia is being used, ask for the qualifications of the anaesthetist or in the US and Canada it may be an anaesthetist nurse. In section two you can find detailed information about anaesthetic options and how to check the qualifications of the practitioner who will administer a general anaesthetic.

4. How many operations do you complete each day, and how many days a week do you operate?

Your plastic surgeon should perform no more than four to six surgical procedures per day.

5. Approximately what percentage of your patients have experienced complications in the past 12 months?

Given that it should be thoroughly documented, responding to this should be straightforward.

6. Have there ever been any patient fatalities or post-surgery needs for acute care or life-saving treatment?

It should be simple to answer this because it should be well documented.

7. What certifications does the clinic or hospital have where I will have my procedure?

Accreditation from a reputable medical organisation is required for hospitals and outpatient surgery centres/clinics.

8. Does the hospital have an Intensive Care Unit?

If the facility does not have an intensive care unit what hospital do you have arrangements with if I needed intensive care? (In the UK part of CQC registration is to have emergency patient facilities in place)

9. Will I incur any additional costs if I need intensive care or ongoing care?

Ask for written confirmation of all associated costs and exactly what is covered following your procedure.

10. If I experience any postoperative issues or don't like the outcomes, will there be any further costs?

It is essential to ask for written confirmation of any additional expenses that may apply in the event of post-operative difficulties or if you are dissatisfied with the results.

"Step into the best version of yourself"

2. THE FUNDAMENTALS

A. SURGICAL AND ANAESTHESIA RISKS AND COMPLICATIONS

Understanding the risks and complications associated with anaesthesia and surgery can be overwhelming - in this section you will find explanations of the most common risks and potential complications associated with cosmetic surgery and anaesthesia that you may experience.

Key Inherent Risks and Complications Associated With Surgical Procedures

Surgical procedures have significantly advanced over the years, however it is crucial to acknowledge that there are inherent risks and potential complications associated with any type of surgery.

The key inherent risks and complications associated with surgical procedures include:

➢ **Anaesthesia:** All surgical procedures will require some form of anaesthetic. This may be general anaesthetic, GA, when you are asleep, or local anaesthetic, LA, where the area being treated is anaesthetised. LA may be combined with some form of sedation, for larger procedures or when patients are anxious.

The risks of any type of anaesthetic are low, particularly as patients undergoing cosmetic surgery do not have significant medical problems. Patients worry about being aware during a general anaesthetic. This is extremely rare and is associated with the use of muscle relaxants, which are rarely required. Issues with allergy to anaesthetics are rare and patients' concerns about not waking up afterwards are exceptionally rare, particularly in a young, fit group.

The research indicates that the risk of dying during pre planned surgery is extremely low if you are in good health. The estimated number of deaths associated with GA is 0.0001% or one death for every 100,000.

Advancements with equipment, training and drugs have made general anaesthesia a safe procedure for most. Cosmetic surgery should only be performed on physically fit people, who are in low risk groups. This significantly reduces the risks associated with a general anaesthetic.

➤ **Scars:** All surgical procedures that involve cutting the skin will leave scars. The quality of the scar left is down to how you heal. In an ideal world all scars would end up as fine white lines, but scars can stretch and they can thicken up; rarely creating keloid scars. Oils and silicone treatments can make scars more comfortable. A specialised cream, <u>Solution for Scars</u>, has been proven to reduce scar thickness, reduce redness, increase scar pliability and improve hydration. Importantly, these benefits in scar outcomes are, further, improved if the cream is used, around the surgical site, for a week in advance of treatment.

➤ **Bleeding:** This can lead to bruising and collections of blood, (haematomas) at the operation site. These may need further surgical intervention to drain and explore the bleeding point. Rapid blood loss from the surgical site may necessitate interventions such as fluid resuscitation and even blood transfusions.

➤ **Seromas:** A collection of fluid under the skin, at the site of a surgical treatment, which can develop soon after surgery or up to two weeks afterward. Small seromas often resolve on their own. However, large seromas may need to be drained. Seromas can sometimes recur and may require multiple drainages. In rare cases, they can become infected or develop into an abscess, which may necessitate treatment.

➢ **Wound infection**: Any cut in the skin risks infection. We are all covered in bacteria which can contaminate the surgical site. To minimise risks, antibiotics may be given over the operative period. If established, infection will be treated with antibiotics and, in severe cases, surgical drainage.

➢ **Deep vein thrombosis (DVT)**: Blood clot formation in a large vein, usually in the legs, which can lead to serious complications such as pulmonary embolism. Prevention includes measures such as compression stockings, calf compression boots, blood thinners and early mobilisation.

➢ **Pulmonary embolism**: A blood clot that travels to the lungs, causing a blockage. Prompt treatment with anticoagulants or thrombolytic therapy may be necessary.

➢ **Urinary retention**: Inability to empty the bladder, which can be caused by anaesthesia or specific surgeries. Catheterisation and medications may be used to manage this complication.

Anaesthesia Options

The two main types of anaesthesia used for cosmetic and plastic surgery are general anaesthetic (GA) and local anaesthetic (LA).

1. General Anaesthesia (GA)

A GA is a state of controlled unconsciousness. To facilitate breathing a breathing tube is inserted and then removed once consciousness begins to return. Throughout the procedure, the anaesthetist carefully monitors and adjusts the depth of anaesthesia for patient safety and comfort, ensuring a controlled and pain free surgical experience.

SIDE EFFECTS OF **GA**:

- Sore throat
- Vomiting and nausea
- Feeling lightheaded and faint.
- Experiencing chills or shivers.
- Headaches.
- Itching
- Difficulty with urination.

2. Local Anaesthesia (LA)

Injected into a specific area of the body, local anaesthetic, also referred to as regional anaesthesia, prevents pain sensation in the targeted region. A peripheral nerve block is the most common type of LA used for cosmetic breast surgery.

Unlike general anaesthesia, it does not induce unconsciousness or loss of awareness, making it a safer option with less side effects. A peripheral nerve block prevents nerve signals in the administered area, which stops pain signals from reaching the brain.

SIDE EFFECTS OF **LA**:

- Vertigo and dizziness
- Headaches
- Impaired vision
- Trembling or twitching muscles

- Itching
- Numbness, weakness, or pins and needles in or around the area injected.

Sedation (with Local Anaesthesia)

Administered into a vein, sedation induces a relaxed state of consciousness, making people feel drowsy. Typically, cardiovascular function is maintained, and individuals are able to breathe independently. Sedation is usually monitored by an anaesthetist or a specially qualified nurse.

There are three levels of sedation, often referred to as twilight sedation, each with its own characteristics:

➢ **Mild:** This level of sedation will help to relax you, you'll remain fully awake and responsive.

➢ **Moderate:** Most commonly used for cosmetic breast surgery, with moderate sedation, you may feel sleepy and drift off during your procedure, but you can easily wake up.

➢ **Deep:** Similar to general anaesthesia, with deep sedation you'll be in a deep sleep.

SIDE EFFECTS OF SEDATION:

- Vomiting and nausea (this can be brought on by the sedative medicine or the surgery)
- Confusion and disorientation.

Benefits of Twilight Sedation

Twilight sedation is regarded as a safer alternative to general anaesthesia due to the patient's sustained consciousness and reactivity to external stimuli. This state of alertness substantially mitigates the probability of encountering medical complications, including respiratory distress or unfavourable pharmacological reactions.

In most cases you can go back home and resume their regular activities a few hours after the surgery. When general anaesthesia is used you may need to stay in the hospital for several hours or possibly overnight for monitoring

Final Thoughts

As you can see, there are many potential risks and complications associated with surgery and anaesthesia. These should be discussed at consultation and you must weigh the potential benefits of your cosmetic breast surgery procedure with a realistic understanding of the associated risks. Choice of anaesthesia will depend on health conditions, patient preference and the procedure, but they all need appropriate management.

The anaesthetist and plastic surgeon you choose can make a vast difference to your surgery's successful outcome, as well as your physical and emotional well being afterwards. Always take the time to make sure you understand all of the associated risks and potential complications of the recommended anaesthetic before undergoing any type of cosmetic or plastic surgery procedure.

Make sure your anaesthetist and plastic surgeon are experienced and properly qualified, and that where your treatment takes place is accredited by appropriate medical bodies, and of high quality. Ask as many questions as necessary and, above all, make sure that you are comfortable with all aspects relating to your surgery, including your expectations being realistically met by what can be done.

Annabelle Baugh, Founder of Cosmetic Surgery Advancements.

B. BREAST AUGMENTATION SURGERY

1. BREAST AUGMENTATION WITH IMPLANTS

In this section, we will provide you with guidance on important considerations regarding your options when it comes to breast augmentation with breast implants. Our aim is to ensure that you can make well informed decisions in collaboration with your plastic surgeon.

Breast Implant Options

Breast implant selection is a complex process that involves considering factors such as implant shapes, sizes, surface textures, and filler attributes. Various implant options are available and correct selection of breast implants will depend on your preferred breast size and shape.

Additional considerations include your natural breast shape, skin elasticity, placement and incision options, which will further impact the final breast shape following augmentation. All of these aspects should be considered to ensure the outcome meets your desired breast shape and size.

When it comes to breast implants, there are several factors to consider; outlined in more detail below. Understanding these differences is crucial in determining the most suitable implants for your physiology, goals, and preferences. Ultimately, the choice of implant size and type should be based on your individual anatomy, aesthetic objectives, and discussions with your plastic surgeon.

Implant Size: Finding the Right Fit

Choosing the right size implant is crucial for achieving your desired results. Breast implant sizers can help you, but, ultimately the final outcome of breast augmentation with implants can not be determined by sizers.

As a general rule, the width of the implant is based on the width of your own breast. Using the full width allows a closer cleavage. However, this will also depend on the surgical technique and skill of your plastic surgeon. The implant projection will influence the degree the implants 'stick out' from your chest wall, and will also affect the fulness achieved in the upper part of your breasts. Other factors aside from the implants selected that will influence the final outcome of your breast augmentation are:

- Density of breast tissue
- Skin elasticity
- Surgical technique and skill
- How well you heal.

Your surgeon should guide you in selecting an implant size, taking into account factors such as your body frame, existing breast tissue, and your personal aesthetic goals. Showing your plastic surgeon photographs of breasts that are as close as possible to the size and shape you would like can be helpful. It is important to communicate your desired outcomeclearly to your plastic surgeon.

Key Information: Saline and Silicone Breast Implants

There are two main types of filler materials for breast implants available: saline and silicone gel. Saline implants consist of a silicone outer shell filled with sterile saltwater. Silicone gel implants have a silicone outer shell filled with a cohesive silicone gel. The consistency of this gel can be varied, to alter the end result.

Saline Breast Implants

Advantages:

- Saline implants allow the plastic surgeon to adjust the volume during your procedure, enabling customisation of size
- Overfilling saline implants is possible when a larger implants size is desired
- Saline implants require smaller incisions and are the only option for transumbilical breast augmentation (T.U.B.A)
- In case of rupture, the saline is harmlessly absorbed by the body.

Disadvantages:

- More prone to rippling which can be noticeable on the surface of the skin
- Weigh more than silicone implants which means they will stretch the skin more over time
- Do not compress as naturally or feel similar to breast tissue

- Some individuals say they feel a strange sensation of the saline 'sloshing' inside the implants
- Higher rates of implant rupture.

Silicone Implants

Advantages:

- Cohesive silicone gel is pliable and mimics the same feel and density as breast tissue
- Only option for teardrop (anatomical) implants which can produce a more natural breast shape for women with little breast tissue
- Lower tendency to ripple or show ripples through the skin, especially in individuals with less breast tissue
- Lower implant rupture rates.

Disadvantages:

- Require a slightly longer incision
- Prefilled and therefore can not be adjusted during the surgical procedure
- If they rupture there is a possibility that silicone gel could migrate into other areas of the body (Gummy bear implants provide an alternative to standard silicone gel and are extremely unlikely to cause silicone migration as they are 'semi solid' similar to a gummy bear).

Implant Volumes

Implant size is determined by volume, which is given in cubic centimetres (cc).

➤ **Silicone breast implants** come in a maximum of 1000cc (pre manufactured).

➤ **Saline breast implants** can be overfilled, however this voids any warranties.

➤ **Silicone and Saline** filled breast implants are available from Mentor's Becker line. These implants feature two distinct lumens (parts). The outer one is prefilled with silicone gel and the internal one is filled with saline during the procedure. This give some degree of customisation and a fill up to 1200cc.

➤ **Tissue expanders**, often referred to as 'expandable implants' contain saline and are filled on the day of the procedure. They can be considered when patients are wanting larger implants. The cc volume can be increased over time by adding extra saline following the procedure. However, most tissue expanders are not considered as long term devices. Ideally they should be changed for permanent implants once the desired breast size has been achieved. Tissue expanders can be overfilled to between 1500cc and 2000cc, however, there are plastic surgeons willing to overfill tissue expanders up to as much as 3000cc.

Implant Dimensions and Shapes

Implant dimensions will impact the shape and size of your breasts and are also determined by your chest width. The three key dimensions are:

1. **Height:** The height of the implant impacts the position, with larger heights resulting in a higher placement on the chest wall.

This typically results in the upper part of the breasts volume starting closer to the collarbone.

2. Width: Implant width should be appropriate to the base width of the patient's own chest wall, with wider implants generally creating a closer and fuller cleavage.

3. Projection: This correlates to the profile of the implants and impacts how much they protrude from the chest wall and the fullness of the upper part of the breasts.

ALTHOUGH IMPLANTS COME IN HUNDREDS, if not thousands of different dimensions there are only two implant shapes:

1. Round (non- anatomical) implants: Depending on the projection, round implants can generate more fullness in the upper breast or a more natural sloping breast shape. High profile round implants are often chosen to produce a fuller and larger breast size. Smaller cc volumes in round implants with low and medium projections can be used to produce a more natural breast shape.

2. Teardrop (anatomical) implants: Certain individuals may require teardrop shaped implants to produce a more natural breast shape. Contoured to resemble the shape of a natural breast, they have less volume in the upper pole and more at the base. As with round implants, teardrop implants are available in a range of widths, heights and projections which will impact the overall shape of the breasts and the amount of volume in the upper breast.

Implant Profiles

Implant profile, (projection), corresponds to how far the implants extend out from your chest wall when you're standing. Profiles available are:

. . .

➤ LOW PROFILE: These have a wider contour and less projection

➤ **Moderate profile:** Offering greater projection than low profile but not as much as high profile implants, moderate profile implants can provide more upper breast volume while still producing a natural breast shape.

➤ **High profile:** These implants tend to create a rounder breast shape and create the highest degree of projection and volume in the upper pole. Generally the higher the profile - the greatest increase in breast size is achieved.

Implant Shell Textures

Breast implants come with silicone exterior shells that can either be smooth or textured:

Textured Implants

Coarse (macro) textured implants, which helped reduce the risk of implant rotation are no longer available, because of their associated risk of BIA-ALCL, (explained below under risks and complications).Currently the two types of implant textures available are micro-textured and meso-textured.

CONSIDERATIONS:

➤ Micro-textured are considered slightly more effective for encouraging tissue growth into the implant's surface helping to prevent implant misplacement

➤ All teardrop implants have a microtextured shell to help reduce the potential for implant rotation or displacement

➤ Textured shells may cause breasts to feel slightly firmer and as the implant secures itself to the capsule can reduce the degree the breasts 'bounces'.

Smooth Implants

Smooth shelled implants have risen in popularity because they are not associated with BIA-ALCL, BIA-SCC or the development of other carcinomas and lymphomas (explained below under risks and complications).

CONSIDERATIONS:
➢ Smooth implants may produce a softer feeling breast
➢ Higher associated rate of capsular contraction, especially with subglandular (above the muscle) placement of smooth implants
➢ An increased associated rate of implant displacement has been linked to smooth implants

Breast Augmentation Surgery Techniques

Breast enlargement procedures are typically performed under general anaesthetic, although some plastic surgeons may use local anaesthetic for primary breast augmentation procedures. The surgery usually lasts between 30 to 60 minutes, depending on the surgeon's technique, implant size and placement options.

Your plastic surgeon and where the procedure is performed, will determine if you have the option to be a day patient or stay in a hospital overnight.

Breast Implant Placement Options

The two most common placement options for breast implants are the
   subglandular and submuscular which are explained below.

1. Subglandular

This placement is above the pectoral muscle and is a popular choice for patients with enough breast tissue to cover the implant fully.

Advantages:

- Generally comes with less painful recovery
- Implants are not impacted by muscle movement
- Contours of breasts are altered more by the actual dimensions of the implants
- Some individuals may prefer the greater projection achieved with non anatomical (round) implants in the top portion of the breasts.

Disadvantages:

- Implant edges may show if there is not much breast tissue present
- Lack of breast tissue or with the use of larger implants increase the potential for viable implant's surface ripples showing beneath the skin
- There may be a higher rate of capsular contracture
- Can cause more interference with mammograms.

1. Breast Augmentation With Implants | 53

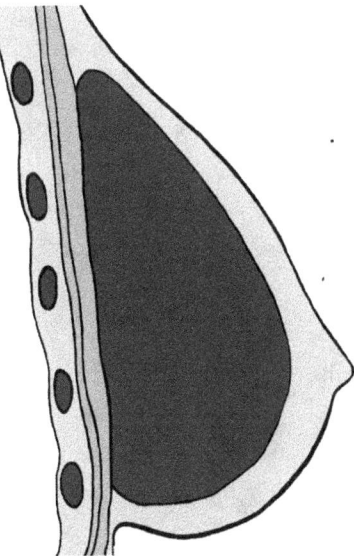

Subglandular Breast Implant Placement

2. Submuscular (Dual Plane)

Submuscular placement is also referred to as dual plane placement, with the upper part of the implants under the pectoral muscle and the lower part exposed.

It is typically preferred to a total submuscular placement for individuals with minimal breast tissue, as it provides many of the advantages, while reducing the problems that are associated with the submuscular placement.

Advantages:

- Lowers the possibility of implant rippling
- Gives the upper breast an additional layer of coverage in the upper part of the breasts that helps to hide the outer edges of implants
- Could decrease the potential of capsular contracture.

Disadvantages:

- Muscle movement means breast implants could be prone to deformity
- Decreases the breast's upper volume, which some individuals might consider a negative.

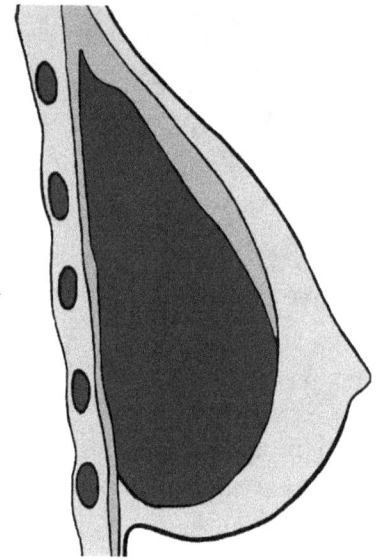

Submuscular (Dual Plane) Breast Implant Placement

Breast Implant Incision Options

Selecting the incision option for breast augmentation is crucial due to its impact on scar location, implant placement, and size and shape limitations. The four options are:

1. Inframammary

The inframammary incision is positioned in the natural crease under the breasts. Suitable for non anatomical (round) and anatomical (teardrop) implants this is the most commonly used incision option. Anatomical (teardrop) implants will normally need to be placed via the inframammary incision as they can not be manipulated to go through a smaller incision.

Advantages:

- Provides optimal access to breast tissue, and allows for more accurate implant placement
- Helps to facilitate the creation of a properly sized pocket for larger silicone implants
- Reduces manipulation of the implants allowing for easier placement of teardrop and larger silicone implants.

Disadvantages:

- Scarring may be visible on or underneath the breasts if the incision is not correctly positioned in the breast crease
- Scarring is generally visible when arms are raised or when lying down.

2. Transaxillary

Positioned in the armpit, the transaxillary incision presents challenges, which can be in part mitigated by using the endoscopic technique. This incision can not be used with teardrop implants and is also less popular than the inframammary and periareolar incision limiting your choice of plastic surgeon.

Advantages:

- Incisions tend to heal faster
- Excellent concealment of scars.

Disadvantages:

- Restricts the size of silicone implants
- Increased potential for implant displacement
- Higher potential of incorrect placement
- Higher risk of capsular contraction
- Potential for infection increases
- Higher risk of bleeding and hematomas
- Might cause damage to the lymphatic and nerves under the arms
- Implants tend to sit higher on the chest which can look unnatural
- Greater possibility for asymmetry.

3. Periareolar

Positioned around the outer bottom edge of the areola in a semi-circle, this incision can be used for round and teardrop implants.

Advantages:

- Good access to breast tissue enabling precise implant placement
- Scars tend to be well hidden by the difference in texture and colour between the areola and the breast skin

- Can be used to lift the breast at the same time as performing breast augmentation.

Disadvantages:

- Potential for highly visible scars if they don't heal well
- Increased risk of infection
- May have a higher potential to cause capsular contraction
- A greater likelihood to damage milk ducts, which can make breastfeeding challenging`
- Increased risk of nerve injury and loss of feeling in and around the nipple.

4. Transumbilical

Referred to as transumbilical breast augmentation (TUBA) this incision is positioned inside the belly button. This procedure can only be performed using saline filled implants, and is not offered by plastic surgeons in the UK.

Advantages:

- Faster recovery and lower pain levels
- Reduced risk of losing nipple sensitivity
- Less risk of complications with larger implants
- Lower risk of infection
- No risk of implant extrusion occurring through the incision.

Disadvantages:

- Tracks created may remain visible in the abdomen
- Higher potential for poor breast shape and asymmetry.

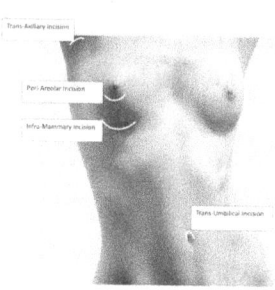

Breast Implant Incisions

Recovery Timeline

Breast implant recovery will vary depending on the placement, incision, surgical technique and individual anatomy. Below is a general guideline to recovery and the time it will take to see the final results.

➢ **Hospital Stay:** In most cases you will be able to return home a few hours after the procedure. Occasionally you may need to stay for one night in hospital, this is more likely if you have had a general anaesthetic or larger implants.

➢ **Recovery time:** Most people are back doing normal day to day activities within one week and you can drive when you feel safe to do so. More rigorous exercises and carrying heavy objects should be avoided for at least six weeks to ensure optimal healing.

You may suffer swelling, bruising, and soreness following surgery, which will subside over the next two to four weeks. Following the surgeon's postoperative care instructions, including wearing support garments, is critical during the healing period.

➢ **Follow up appointments:** At least one follow up appointment should take place approximately 10 to 14 days after the procedure. Typically sutures are dissolvable, although sometimes they will not dissolve completely and sometimes sutures may need to be removed at this appointment.

➢ **Time until results:** Although the results of a breast augmentation are immediately visible, as the skin stretches to its natural tension, and the breast implants settle into their new position, breast shape will alter over a three to six month period

Final results are normally apparent within six months, however, breast shape may continue to change subtly over the course of the first 12 months following breast augmentation. Breasts will continue to sag over time and depending on the implant size, placement option and individual anatomy, this may be anything from a subtle to a more severe drop.

Risks and Complications

Breast augmentation carries the same risks associated with all surgical procedures.

In addition there are risks and complications that are associated only with breast augmentation with implants.

Common Risks and Complications

➤ **Capsular contraction:** All implants form a scar capsule around them. As this scar matures, it can shrink, resulting in breast firmness or hardening and a rounder breast shape. This is called capsular contraction and can cause persistent pain and result in implant displacement. It's a limitation of healing and impacts the quality of result achieved in a relatively small proportion of patients.

➤ **Haematoma and Seroma:** Haematomas and seromas are collections of fluid (seromas) or blood (haematomas) around the breast implant. They have the potential to produce swelling, discomfort, and bruising. Small seromas and haematomas can be absorbed by the body, but larger ones may require a surgical drain.

➤ **Sensation:** Breast augmentation can interfere with skin and nipple sensation, although this tends to be temporary it can be permanent.

➤ **Rippling and visible edges:** Breast implants might fold or wrinkle which can be felt under the skin. Rippling is more of a problem with saline breast implants, which are more fluid than silicone implants. Breast implant edges and apparent ripples are also more apparent when there is a lack of breast tissue and thin skin. This may be the reason you have been advised to have a submuscular, dual plane placement.

➤ **Rupture:** Both silicone and saline breast implants can rupture. This is commonly associated with capsular contraction. When a saline breast implant ruptures, the saline is simply absorbed. Rupture of a silicone breast implant is often not noticeable and the silicone may migrate and result in inflammatory lumps, (siliconomas), or enlarged lymph nodes.

Causes of breast implant rupture include:

- External injury to the breast

- Capsular contraction
- Incorrectly sized pocket resulting in the implants wrinkling or folding
- Breast implants of poor quality
- Breast implants that are damaged during surgery.

➢ **Misplacement issues:** If the pocket made for the implant is too large or poorly placed, breast implants may not sit as anticipated. Careful pocket placement is even more important now that coarse (macro) textured implant surfaces are no longer used. In addition it is important that there is proper support to prevent implant displacement.

Breast augmentation does not treat drooping of the breast, (ptosis). Placing an implant low, to disguise a droop can lead to a double bubble deformity, where the original inferior breast fold creates a groove across the breast. Breast implants can displace, under the influence of gravity, and it is important to consider the quality of the tissues in choosing implant size. Larger implants are more likely to stretch the breast skin and suffer with misplacement issues..

➢ **Symmastia:** Breast implants that are placed to close together, may damage the cleavage, giving the appearance of breasts that unite in the middle of the chest, referred to as symmastia. This can be difficult to treat. A shallow cleavage can occur naturally and should be identified and discussed in advance of surgery.

Rare Risks and Complications

➢ **Infection:** Infection can occur after any surgical procedure. Infection around breast implants is rare and antibiotics may be given over the operative period to minimise the risk. In most cases infections are successfully treated with antibiotics, occasionally this may be via an intravenous antibiotic drip.

When an infection does not respond to antibiotics, implant removal may be necessary. Typically the implants can be replaced within three to six months after the infection has cleared up.

➢ **Scarring:** Inserting implants requires creating an incision which will scar. The quality of the scar will depend on surgical technique and on how you heal. Most scars will be fine and pale, but some scars may stretch and thicken. Rarely, this can develop into a bulky scar that extends beyond the original skin injury; called a keloid scar.

It is important to inform your surgeon if you know that you have a tendency for keloid scars so that appropriate measures can be taken to minimise the risk of keloid formation. Using Solution for Scars can help to improve scar outcomes and should also be used in advance of surgery for the best results.

➢ **Implant extrusion:** Breast implant extrusion occurs when the implant protrudes through the skin after breast augmentation, usually from breakdown of the scar. Causes of this are normally thin skin, poor quality tissues, oversized implants, and, or infection. If extrusion occurs or is at risk, it is highly likely that the implants will be removed. Implants are generally replaced (if desired) within a three to six month period.

➢ **Necrosis:** The development of dead skin or tissue around the breast is known as necrosis. It is rare with breast augmentation but can be an issue if skin tightening and reshaping procedures are done at the same time. Smoking raises the risk of necrosis and should be stopped at least six weeks in advance of surgery.

➢ **Breast implant associated – anaplastic large cell lymphoma (BIA-ALCL):** BIA-ALCL is linked to textured implants and currently, there is no correlation between BIA-ALCL with individuals who have solely received smooth shelled implants. The possibility of developing BIA-ALCL is still under debate, however, evidence from credible sources indicates that fewer than 0.1% of individuals with textured implants are diagnosed with the condition. Given that, though the risk of BIA-ALCL is low, it is essential it is identified and treated in a timely manner. Both silicone and saline-filled implants have been linked to BIA-ALCL.

➢ **Breast implant associated – squamous cell carcinoma (BIA-SCC) and other lymphomas** : The potential risk of BIA-SCC and other types of carcinomas and lymphomas is considered extremely low. These very rare lymphomas have been linked to both saline and silicone-filled implants, as well as smooth and textured implant shells.

The FDA received 24 medical device reports (MDRs) about SCC and breast implants as of January 15, 2023, according to the most recent FDA update, released on March 8, 2023. Currently, there is no correlation between BIA-SCC and other carcinomas or lymphomas, in individuals who have only ever had smooth shelled implants.

Eight Key Things to Ask About Breast Augmentation Surgery

1. Experience and risks and complications

Ask your plastic surgeon how many times they have carried out this kind of procedure over the past three months. Discuss the potential risks and complications, as well as asking about how often these have occurred and how they were resolved.

2. Facility

Ask where your surgery will take place and check certifications - refer to Section One - Regulatory Medical Bodies, for more information about facility certifications.

3. Anaesthesia

Breast augmentation with implants is generally performed under a general anaesthetic. However, some plastic surgeons may perform this procedure using a localised anaesthetic and intravenous sedation. Ask which anaesthesia options are available and the advantages and disadvantages of each kind.

4. Breast Implant Questions

➢ **Volume:** Inquire about the various implant volumes and ask your plastic surgeon to explain their recommendations based on your specific goals and body type.

➢ **Shape and profile:** Discuss the options and how the shape and profile will impact breast shape and the final outcome.

➢ **Height and width:** Ask for your chest width measurements and how the recommended width and height of your implants will impact how they sit on your chest wall and your cleavage.

➢ **Incision and placement:** Inquire about the various incision locations and implant placement options, as well as the surgeon's recommendations for your desired result and body type.

5. Risks and complications

Which are the most frequent problems or complications you have had with this surgery, and how did you address them?

6. Revision surgery

Ask if there are any charges for revision surgery, if there is a complication or you are not happy with the results. (Confirmation of the cost of additional revision surgery including any additional hospital or anaesthetist costs, and exactly what is covered should be provided in writing.)

7. Implant warranty

Check what type of warranty is provided with the implant and what you would need to do to male a claim if it was to rupture or found to be defective.

8. Recovery expectations

Find out about the recovery process, including downtime, post operative care and how you can contact your plastic surgeon or receive medical care if you have any concerns.

Breast Implant FAQ

1. **What is the lifespan of breast implants?**

Nowadays, breast implants frequently include a lifetime warranty. Breast implants were once thought to last ten years, but the more recent silicone breast implants have changed this. However, saline breast implants are more prone to rupture and will require replacement sooner.

2. **Can breast implants cause breast cancer?**

Numerous clinical investigations have been done to determine whether there is a link between breast implants and breast cancer. The results indicate that there is no increased risk of breast cancer in individuals with implants. However, implants can shadow the breast tissue in standard view mammograms and specialist views should be taken.

3. **What is breast implant associated anaplastic large cell lymphoma (BIA-ALCL)?**

BIA-ALCL is a rare form of lymphatic cancer that has been linked to implants with a coarse textured shell, referred to as macro textured. The textured shell triggers a reaction and cancerous cells develop in the scar capsule around the implant. Allergan withdrew their range of highly textured biocell implants in July 2019 which have the highest associated rate of diagnosed cases of BIA-ALCL. Many other implant companies have since withdrawn certain styles of textured implants.

The risk of developing BIA-ALCL is extremely low and is currently estimated between 0.01% and 0.1% according to clinical studies. Diagnosis is relatively straightforward and most patients are successfully treated with complete removal of the scar capsule along with the implants; called an en bloc capsulectomy. In rare cases, when not detected early enough, patients may require subsequent treatments such as chemotherapy, radiotherapy, and additional surgery.

4. **Do breast implants affect mammograms?**

According to the FDA, breast implants conceal breast tissue by between 22% and 83% in mammography scans. Breast implants filled with silicone and saline have both been known to rupture as a result of mammography, although this is considered rare. Subsequently it's critical to inform your doctor and the radiographer if you have implants so that special techniques can be used.

5. Can you breastfeed with implants?

Most women are still able to breastfeed following breast augmentation.

Breast implants placed through a periareolar incision may make it difficult to breastfeed as, during the surgery some of the milk ducts are divided.

Final Thoughts

The overall appearance and feel of breast implants can differ depending on the individual. Choosing the right implants and surgical options that meet your individual preferences for breast augmentation, requires thorough research and asking the right questions. The best person who can guide you about your surgical options and help you choose the best implants for your individual anatomy and preferences is your plastic surgeon.

Annabelle Baugh, Founder of Cosmetic Surgery Advancements

2. AUTOLOGOUS BREAST FAT TRANSFER

New techniques and advancements with fat transfer means it is now possible to have bigger, fuller breasts without the need for implants. This procedure involves removing excess fat from areas like the hips, abdomen, lower back, or thighs using liposuction. Then, the extracted fat is skillfully injected into your breasts, strategically enhancing them without the use of implants. It's done as an outpatient procedure, meaning you can go home the same day.

Not only does this procedure give you larger breasts, it also has the added benefit of improving your body contours by reducing fat in other areas, and the best part is that there is minimal scarring. Size increase is limited and treatment may require more than one procedure. Not all injected fat will survive and revisions may be necessary. Fat injection should be done by a properly trained plastic surgeon so that long term potential problems with breast screening are minimised.

Whilst there are issues using autologous fat this technique can offer advantages for selected patients.The results may look and feel more natural, and it avoids the complications associated with implants such as implant rupture, or capsular contraction.

Fat transfer, also referred to as autologous fat injections, is a technique for breast augmentation that has increased steadily in popularity since the 1900's. Aside from its application in numerous surgical areas, fat transfer is widely utilised in the field of breast surgery for both aesthetic and reconstructive objectives. Whilst size increases are modest, fat transfer may be suitable for small augmentations and the correction of some asymmetries.

As the use of fat tissue transplantation in breast surgery has grown in popularity, likewise has research examining the efficacy of this procedure. Fat grafting has been an established technique used by plastic surgeons to enhance and improve the physical appearance of the face, breasts, buttocks and other areas of the body, <u>since the 1990s</u>.

Furthermore, medical professionals have provided evidence of the beneficial effects of grafting fat with regard to the repair of burns wounds and to improve scars, and they have additionally demonstrated the capacity of <u>fat for repairing compromised breast tissue</u> after radiation therapy.

Autologous Breast Augmentation Procedure

Autologous breast fat transfer procedures are frequently carried out on a day case basis, utilising local anaesthesia, although general anaesthesia may be used if preferred by the surgeon or patient.The entire process, which includes liposuction, typically takes between one to three hours. Below is an outline of the procedure:

➢ **Donor site selection:** The selection of a suitable donor site is a crucial step in the fat transfer procedure. Common donor areas include the abdomen, thighs, or buttocks, where there is an ample supply of excess adipose tissue. The surgeon carefully evaluates these areas based on the patient's anatomy and desired outcome.

➢ **Liposuction harvesting:** Before the liposuction procedure, the chosen donor area is infiltrated with a local anaesthetic to minimise discomfort. Liposuction involves the insertion of a thin tube, called a cannula, through small incisions in the skin. The surgeon carefully manoeuvres the cannula to suction out excess fat deposits. The goal is to harvest fat cells while preserving their viability for transfer.

Specialised liposuction techniques, such as power-assisted liposuction (PAL) or ultrasound-assisted liposuction (UAL), may be employed to enhance the precision and effectiveness of fat removal. These techniques help maintain the integrity of fat cells for optimal survival during the transfer process.

➤ **Fat Processing:** Once the fat is harvested, it undergoes a processing phase to purify it before injection. The harvested fat is typically treated to remove impurities such as blood, oil, and other fluids. This purification step is crucial for enhancing the survival rate of the transferred fat cells.

The purified fat is then carefully prepared for injection. The processing phase may involve centrifugation or filtration techniques to separate the healthy fat cells from unwanted substances.

➤ **Fat transfer:** The surgeon strategically places multiple small incisions on the breast. These incisions are strategically placed to minimise scarring and are often located in inconspicuous areas. The fat is injected in small, carefully measured amounts using small plastic cannulas (tubes), to create the desired shape and volume. Absorbable sutures or surgical adhesive are used to close the incisions.

OVERALL, the success of autologous breast augmentation relies on the plastic surgeon's skill and expertise in each phase of the procedure; from donor site selection to precise fat injection and incision closure. You should always have a consultation with your plastic surgeon prior to the procedure, to understand the specific techniques that will be employed based on your unique anatomy and goals.

Autologous Breast Augmentation vs Breast Implants

Advantages

- **Natural look and feel:** Transferred fat typically feels and appears the same as natural breast tissue.
- **Minimal visible scars:** The procedure involves small incisions, leaving you with minimal scarring.
- **No implant complications:** Unlike breast augmentation with implants, this procedure avoids complications such as skin thinning, capsular contraction, and implant rupture or displacement.

Disadvantages and Limitations

- **Limited suitability:** Individuals who smoke or who want to lose weight or have fluctuating weight changes might not be suitable candidates.
- **Moderate increase in cup size:** While this procedure can provide an enhancement, the increase in cup size is typically limited to one or two sizes.
- **Possibility of multiple procedures:** Depending on your desired results, you may need more than one procedure to achieve your goals.
- **No guaranteed results:** Results can vary from person to person, and individual outcomes may not always match expectations.
- **Fat absorption, and lumps:** Some of the transferred fat may be reabsorbed by the body, resulting in

unsymmetrical breast size and shape, and there are increasing reports of cystic lumps and fat necrosis which causes small hard calcified lumps to form, which could be mistaken for cancerous growths.
- **Regular monitoring:** It's recommended to undergo a yearly ultrasound to monitor any changes in the breast tissue.

Recovery Timeline

Recovery after autologous breast augmentation is generally less invasive than traditional breast implant surgery, but it still requires proper care and attention to ensure a smooth healing process. Here is an overview of the recovery period for autologous breast augmentation:

➢ **Hospital Stay:** Autologous breast augmentation is normally performed on a day case basis, meaning patients can go home on the same day as the surgery.

➢ **Recovery time:** Some discomfort, swelling, and bruising are normal in the first few days and you should take it easy during the first week, avoiding strenuous activities and heavy lifting.

You may be required to wear compression garments to reduce swelling and provide support. Strenuous exercises and activities should be avoided for at least two to six weeks, depending on the surgeon's recommendations.

➢ **Follow up appointments:** At least one follow up appointment should take place approximately 10 to 14 days after the procedure. It's common for additional fat transfer procedures to be required to achieve the size and shape desired. Subsequent fat transfer procedures can typically be performed after three to six months.

➢ **Time until results:** Swelling and bruising should gradually subside over the first two weeks. The full results of autologous breast augmentation may take up to six months to become apparent as the body may absorb some of the transferred fat.

It is essential for patients to closely follow their surgeon's postoperative care instructions and attend all scheduled follow up appointments to ensure a successful and smooth recovery process. Every individual's recovery experience may vary, and consulting with a qualified and experienced plastic surgeon is crucial to achieving the desired outcomes with autologous breast augmentation.

Risks and Complications

Common Risks and Complications

Breast fat transfer, also known as autologous fat grafting, is generally considered a safe and effective procedure, but like any surgery, it comes with its own set of risks and complications. It's important for individuals considering breast fat transfer to be aware of these potential issues:

➢ **Infection:** Any surgical procedure carries the risk of infection. In breast fat transfer, infection can occur at the donor liposuction site (where the fat is harvested) or the recipient site (where the fat is injected into the breasts). Antibiotics are typically prescribed to minimise this risk.

➢ **Fat absorption:** Not all the transferred fat may survive in its new location. Some of the fat cells may be reabsorbed by the body, leading to a reduction in the desired volume or asymmetry. This can result in the need for additional procedures to achieve the desired outcome.

➢ **Cysts:** The development of cysts in the breast tissue is another potential complication. These cysts may be fluid filled and can cause discomfort. They will normally resolve without treatment but may occasionally require treatment with needle aspiration and antibiotics.

➢ **Calcification:** In some cases, calcification may occur following breast augmentation with autologous fat Injection. This can cause firm lumps which necessitate further evaluation through imaging tests, such as mammograms, and biopsies to rule out any concerns.

Rare Risks and Complications

➢ **Seroma formation:** The accumulation of fluid in the operated area, known as a seroma, is a potential complication. A needle aspiration may be necessary for substantial seromas, particularly if they are causing a great deal of pain or swelling.

➢ **Hematoma formation:** A hematoma is a collection of blood that has escaped from blood vessels and accumulated outside the blood vessels, usually within a tissue. Large hematomas may need aspiration with a needle, especially if the hematoma is causing significant pain or swelling.

➢ **Changes in sensation:** Some patients may experience changes in nipple or breast sensation after the procedure. This can range from increased sensitivity to temporary numbness. In most cases, sensation returns to normal over time, but there may be areas of the breast or liposuction sites that remain numb permanently.

➢ **Scarring:** The liposuction incisions made to harvest the fat and the incisions required to inject the transferred fat into the breasts are typically small, but scarring is still a possibility. Proper wound care and adherence to post operative instructions can help minimise scarring.

. . .

PATIENTS WITH A FAMILY history of breast cancer should not undergo autologous breast augmentation since calcifications in the breast parenchyma can be expected and will require investigations to check they are benign. A thorough understanding of the procedure and realistic expectations can help patients make informed decisions and ensure a smoother recovery process.

Four Key Questions to Ask About Autologous Breast Augmentation

If you're considering this procedure, it's crucial to choose an experienced plastic surgeon. Before making your decision, ask:

1. How many autologous fat grafting procedures have you performed in the past 12 months?
2. What is the most common complication you have encountered and how was it rectified?
3. Are there any additional charges for treating complications or asymmetry?
4. What is the largest cup size increase I can expect after one fat transfer procedure?
5. What is the cost for additional procedures to increase size and volume?

Autologous Breast Augmentation FAQ

1. How long does autologous breast augmentation last?

The longevity of autologous breast augmentation, or fat transfer to the breasts may vary among individuals. Factors such as lifestyle, weight fluctuations, and the body's natural ageing process can influence the duration of the results. Generally, a significant portion of the transferred fat will remain in the breasts, but additional procedures may be recommended to maintain or adjust the results over time.

2. Can fat transfer in breasts affect mammograms?

Fat transfer to the breasts can potentially impact the accuracy of mammograms. The injected fat cells may create calcifications that can resemble suspicious findings on mammograms. While skilled radiologists are trained to differentiate between these calcifications and potential signs of breast cancer, it's essential to inform your healthcare provider about the fat transfer procedure before undergoing mammography. Additional imaging techniques or more frequent monitoring may be suggested to ensure accurate breast cancer screening.

3. Can you breastfeed after autologous breast augmentation?

Autologous breast augmentation is not likely to interfere with breastfeeding. However, individual experiences may vary, and it's advisable to discuss your plans for breastfeeding with your plastic surgeon during the consultation to address any specific concerns related to your anatomy and the surgical technique used.

Final Thoughts

Breast augmentation utilising fat transfer is certainly an alternative to implants if you only desire a small increase in breast size and fullness. However, due to the risks of uneven fat absorption, calcified lumps and other complications I would be very cautious of proceeding with fat transfer for the purpose of breast augmentation.

Annabelle Baugh, Founder of Cosmetic Surgery Advancements

3. BREAST IMPLANT ILLNESS (BII), BREAST IMPLANT ASSOCIATED LARGE CELL LYMPHOMA (BIA-ALCL) AND BREAST IMPLANT ASSOCIATED SQUAMOUS CELL CARCINOMA (BIA-SCC)

The safety of breast implants and breast implant illness (BII) has long been a contentious issue. Shortly after silicone filled breast implants became publicly available in the US, women started to report a broad spectrum of health issues, blamed on implants.

Adverse events, including hardening, pain and distortion of implant shape, from capsular contracture and rupture were known limitations with breast implants, but patients complained of multiple other symptoms and a potential connection to autoimmune disease from silicone filled implants.

This led to a significant class action lawsuit in the USA. The FDA, in 1992, introduced a "voluntary moratorium" on silicone breast implants, restricting silicone filled devices to breast reconstruction or replacement of faulty implants. There were limitations on the use of silicone breast implants by the rest of the world.

Following extensive research into silicone filled breast implants and reported health concerns, the FDA found no conclusive evidence that linked the insertion of silicone implants to any of the reported illnesses., It is important to note that oili cone filled implants were never banned in the US, they were under restrictions of use. In 2006 the FDA lifted all limitations on use, due to insufficient proof of any associated health issues.

BII is a term used to refer to a variety of illnesses that people with breast implants have reported being affected with which include:

- Dermatological (skin) issues,
- Pain in the muscles and joints,
- Exhaustion and fatigue
- Concentration problems
- Headaches
- Hair loss.

Scientific evidence linking breast implants to these symptoms or autoimmune disease is contradictory. The current data available indicates that the same symptoms occur in similar incidences in people who do not have silicone implants. Although, in some cases, people have reported improvement in symptoms following implant removal, there is a lack of scientific studies that provide evidence of autoimmune disease or conditions that can be definitively linked to silicone breast implants.

Breast Implant Associated Large Cell Lymphoma (BIA–ALCL)

Breast implant-associated anaplastic large cell lymphoma (BIA-ALCL) a rare type of non-Hodgkin's lymphoma associated with textured breast implants. It is not breast cancer but a lymphoma that can develop in the scar tissue surrounding the implant.

Breast Implants and BIA-ALCL

BIA-ALCL has been associated almost exclusively with textured implants. In particular, there is a higher associated risk between

Allergan's BIOCELL textured breast implants and BIA-ALCL cases. As a result, Allergan withdrew BIOCELL textured implants and tissue expanders from the market, globally, in July 2019.

Other manufacturers of textured implants have also been linked to BIA-ALCL in lower numbers and both silicone and saline filled textured breast implants have been implicated. BIA-ALCL is rare and the regulatory bodies in the UK (MHRA), US/Canada (FDA), Australia (TGA) do not currently recommend routine removal of textured implants. The advice is to monitor for BIA-ALCL symptoms including:

- Swelling or pain
- Lumps
- Skin alterations
- Alterations to breast form.

The majority of patients diagnosed with BIA-ALCL are effectively treated with an en bloc capsulectomy, which involves removing the complete scar capsule and implants in one piece. This is not always possible if the implants have adhered to the chest wall and, or ribs or the scar capsule is not thick enough. Very occasionally, individuals who can not have an en bloc capsulectomy or are not treated promptly enough may need further chemotherapy, radiotherapy and, or surgical procedures..

The risk of developing BIA-ALCL is currently disputed, however according to data from reputable organisations the percentage rate of BIA-ALCL diagnosis is less than 0.1%. According to the most 2020 investigation conducted by the Scientific Committee on Health, Environmental and Emerging Risks (SCHEER), the estimated lifetime incidence varies between 1.65 and 35 cases per 100,000 *(0.00165% and 0.035%).

According to the information as of March 2024 on the American Society of Plastic Surgeons (ASPS) website, the projected lifetime risk of BIA-ALCL is 1:2,207-1:86,029 *(0.045% to 0.001%)

for textured implants over the previous 20 years. Whilst minimal, this risk is present and BIA-ALCL can cause fatality if not diagnosed and treated early enough. To date diagnosis of BIA-ALCL is not associated with individuals who have only ever had smooth shelled implants.

Below are two images to show where the lymphoma cells caused by BIA-ALCL are located in comparison to breast cancer cells.

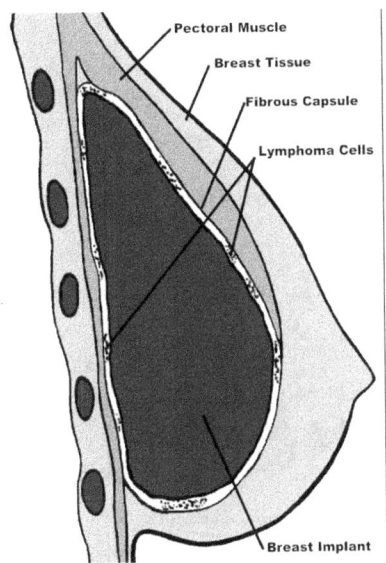

BIA-ALCL Lymphoma Cells

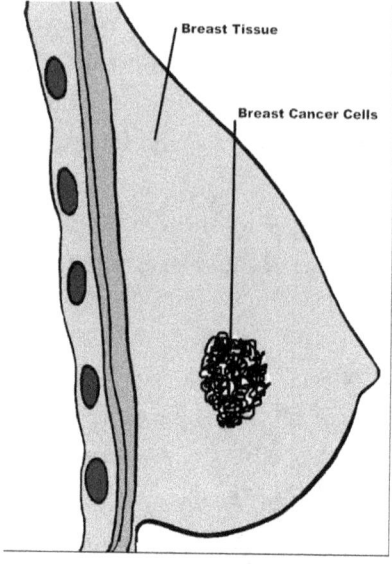

Breast Cancer Cells

Breast Implant Associated Squamous Cell Carcinoma (BIA-SCC)

THERE HAS ONLY BEEN one FDA communication aside from BIA-ALCL regarding a link between cancerous tumours and breast implants. Released on the 8th September 2022 by the US Food and Drug Administration (FDA) a safety <u>communication included reports of squamous cell carcinoma (SCC)</u> and various lymphomas found in the capsule of scar tissue that encompasses breast implants.

These lymphomas are extremely rare and have been connected to textured and smooth implant shells, and both saline and silicone filled implants.In the most recent <u>FDA update on the 8th March 2023</u>, the FDA has been provided with 24 medical device reports (MDRs) about SCC with breast implants as of January 15, 2023.

Breast Implants and Cancer

Breast implants have not been linked to an elevated rate of breast cancer. Interestingly there is data that patients with breast implants have a lower incidence of breast cancer than the general population. This could be interpreted that breast implants help protect women against breast cancer but we know that patients with large fatty breasts have a higher incidence of breast cancer and augmentation is, therefore, being performed in a lower incidence group.

BII and BIA-ALCL FAQ

1. What is Breast Implant Illness (BII)?

Breast Implant Illness refers to a set of symptoms that some individuals with breast implants report, including fatigue, joint pain, and cognitive issues. It's important to note that BII is not a universally recognized medical diagnosis and these symptoms can be caused by numerous health conditions.

2. What is Breast Implant-Associated Anaplastic Large Cell Lymphoma (BIA-ALCL)?

BIA-ALCL, recognized by the World Health Organization (WHO), is a form of non-Hodgkin's lymphoma associated with textured breast implants, often developing within the scar tissue surrounding the implant. While it is considered an official medical diagnosis for cancer, it's crucial to emphasise that the risk of BIA-ALCL is generally very low. However, this risk may vary based on factors such as the type and texture of the implant used.

3. Are certain types of breast implants more associated with BIA-ALCL?

Textured breast implants from various manufacturers have been associated with a higher risk of BIA-ALCL. Some of the manufacturers whose textured implants have been linked to BIA-ALCL include:

- **Allergan** (acquired by AbbVie): Biocell textured implants and Natrelle textured implants have the highest association with diagnosed BIA-ALCL cases.
- **Mentor** (acquired by Johnson & Johnson): MemoryGel™ SILTEX silicone implants
- **Sientra:** Opus™ silicone breast implants
- **GC Aesthetics:** Eurosilicone and Nagor, textured surface silicone breast implants
- **Silimed:** BIODESIGN™ textured surface silicone breast implants
- **Polytech Silimed Europe GmbH:** textured surface silicone breast implants.

THE TGA in Australia has also withdrawn the below implants:

- **Polytech Health & Aesthetics GmbH:** Sublime Line, Microthane silicone breast implants and 4Two Line, Single Lumen, Micro Polyurethane, silicone breast implants
- **Eurosilicone SAS:** Cristaline Paragel Cohesive Gel Implant.

NB: It's important to note that the information regarding associations between manufacturers and BIA-ALCL may evolve, and regulatory agencies continue to monitor and update safety information. For the most current and accurate information, individuals should consult with their healthcare providers and stay informed about updates from regulatory bodies or relevant health authorities in their country.

Final Thoughts

The research and data are always being updated in relation to the various health conditions and illnesses that are thought to be associated with breast implants. Although there is no direct evidence that breast implants have the potential to cause BII it does seem apparent that some women do experience problems that resolve once their implants have been removed. The risk of BIA-ALCL is present but extremely low and studies indicate it to be highest with macro textured breast implants, which are no longer used.It's best to consult a physician if you have any concerns regarding BII symptoms in order to rule out any other underlying reasons. Consult a plastic surgeon about implants removal or replacement if you have concerns regarding BIA-ALCL.

Annabelle Baugh, Founder of Cosmetic Surgery Advancements

4. MONITORING BREAST IMPLANTS FOR RUPTURE

Breast implant rupture is a potential complication that increases with time and is associated with capsular contraction. Implants can't shrink so fold, creating the potential for attrition rupture at the fold point. The most common cause of early breast implant rupture is instrument damage during placement, emphasising the importance of selecting an accredited plastic surgeon. With saline filled implants, the valve at the injection port can fail, allowing leakage and deflation.

Saline Implant Rupture

Saline implants became popular following the FDA restrictions on the use of silicone implants. One of the key reasons was the body's ability to safely absorb and eliminate the saline water if the implant ruptured. The injection valve, though, fails in 2-3% of implants per year.

Signs of Rupture with Saline Implants

When a saline implant ruptures the saline will leak out within a relatively fast period of time and signs of rupture will be evident almost immediately, these include:

- Change in breast shape
- Deflation of breast size
- Reduced firmness of the breast.

Silicone Implant Rupture

Silicone breast implants are the most used and popular implants with both patients and plastic surgeons, for good reason. When compared to failure rates of saline implants, silicone implants are more durable, longer lasting, and widely considered to produce more pleasing aesthetic results, with a more natural feel and look. They have been used for cosmetic and reconstructive purposes for nearly six decades, and they have evolved significantly in design and manufacture, making them, now, more resilient and stable, with lower incidences of capsular contraction.

While they have been subject to intense scrutiny regarding safety, the current generations of silicone implants have been through numerous long term clinical studies and are considered extremely safe. That being said, one of the critical patient concerns associated with them is rupture, which, unlike saline implants, may not always present with noticeable symptoms, commonly referred to as silent rupture.

Signs of Rupture with Silicone Breast Implants

A silent rupture may cause no signs. Modern breast implants contain highly cohesive silicone gel that is normally contained within the scar capsule that is formed around the implant. This is an intracapsular rupture. When the silicone gel migrates outside of the scar capsule this is known as extracapsular rupture and may cause clinical signs that your silicone implant has ruptured including:

- Changes in breast shape and size.
- Ripples under the surface of the skin
- Decreased breast firmness
- Capsular contracture causing breasts to feel firmer
- Skin looks red
- Soreness, pain, burning sensation
- Swelling
- Hard lumps in or near the breast and armpit
- Enlarged lymph nodes.

Tests for Detecting Silent Rupture with Silicone Breast Implants

Clinical studies indicate that detection of implant rupture is challenging because the majority of silicone implant ruptures are undetectable without using one of the scanning modalities.

The two types of scanning are normally used to detect rupture, ultrasound and magnetic resonance imaging (MRI). If you are concerned about rupture, understanding the advantages and disadvantages of each scan can be helpful to aid in an informed decision making process.

Ultrasound for Monitoring Silicone Breast Implant Rupture

Ultrasound is the most commonly used tool to assess silicone breast implants for rupture.

Advantages of Ultrasound

- **Real time imaging:** Provides immediate feedback, allowing immediate visualisation of the implant and surrounding structures.
- **Cost effective:** Compared to MRI, ultrasound is generally more affordable, making it accessible to a broader range of patients.

Disadvantages of Ultrasound

- **Limited sensitivity:** Ultrasound may not detect early stages of implant rupture, particularly in cases of intracapsular rupture where the silicone remains confined to the fibrous capsule.
- **Operator dependent:** The quality of ultrasound images heavily depends on the skills and expertise of the operator, potentially affecting the accuracy of diagnosis.
- **Reduced visualisation:** Ultrasound may have limited visibility in patients with dense breast tissue, hindering accurate assessment in some cases.

MRI for Monitoring Silicone Breast Implant Rupture

Used less frequently than ultrasound, MRI scans are considered particularly effective in detecting both intracapsular and extracapsular rupture.

Advantages of MRI

- **High sensitivity and specificity:** MRI scans have high spatial resolution and show excellent contrast between implants and soft tissues, making it more reliable for early detection.
- **Multi-planar imaging:** This allows imaging in multiple planes, enabling a comprehensive evaluation of the implant and surrounding tissues.
- **Precise Localization:** MRI imaging can more accurately determine whether implant rupture is confined to the capsule or has migrated into breast tissue.

Disadvantages of MRI

- **Cost and accessibility:** MRI scans are generally more expensive than ultrasound and may not be as readily available in all healthcare settings.
- **Claustrophobia and patient comfort:** Some patients may experience claustrophobia or discomfort during MRI scans, potentially leading to suboptimal imaging quality.

Breast Implant Rupture FAQ

1. **How difficult is it to rupture a silicone breast implant?**

Rupture of silicone implants has been associated with injuries that result in an object penetrating the breast or accidents that subject the breast to extreme pressure.

2. **Can ruptured saline implants remain in place?**

The silicone shell containing the saline can be left, but the implant will have lost its volume. In order to contribute to a simpler surgical procedure and quicker recuperation, it is recommended to replace ruptured saline implants as quickly as you can.

3. If a silicone implant ruptures and is not taken out, what are the consequences?

Removing ruptured silicone implants is important if you are experiencing any signs or symptoms of a rupture. Although it is unlikely silicone gel in modern implants will migrate outside of the scar capsule, removal of the implant will prevent this, and therefore is also advisable in the case of a silent rupture in non symptomatic patients.

Final Thoughts

Monitoring silicone breast implants for silent rupture can provide peace of mind. Both ultrasound and MRI play vital roles in this process. MRI is considered the best for detecting implant failure, with high accuracy and sensitivity, especially for patients with dense breast tissue. Discussion with your plastic surgeon will assist in deciding which is best for you.

Staying informed and making evidence based decisions, and, if you are concerned, regular monitoring of your silicone breast implants, can be beneficial to feeling confident and happy.

Annabelle Baugh, Founder of Cosmetic Surgery Advancements

5. BREAST IMPLANT REVISION, REMOVAL OR IMPLANT REPLACEMENT SURGERY

The motivations prompting individuals to choose implant removal followed by replacement, or, in some cases, just implant removal surgery are diverse. Breast implants are not regarded as lifetime devices and as such may sometimes need to be removed or replaced. This could be as a result of implant failure (rupture) or issues such as capsular contraction.

Following breast augmentation with implants, your breasts will change in size and shape over the years. This may result in a desire to have your implants replaced to improve the shape or, and alter the size of your breasts. The treatment journey may involve altering the implant's placement, coupled with techniques such as breast uplift and reshaping, to ensure outcomes that are both optimal and aesthetically pleasing. In instances where a mastopexy (breast uplift) is deemed beneficial, additional surgical expertise is required.

The decision to undergo implant removal without replacement can additionally stem from a range of reasons, encompassing shifts in personal preferences, changing lifestyle choices, and even medical considerations. You may also have concerns about the potential effects of breast implants on your overall health. Additionally, regulatory bodies have recommended removal of certain implant types, including hydrogel, (trilucent) soya filled implants and Poly Implant Prothèse (PIP) implants.

For any or all of these reasons implant removal or replacement might be an option you choose to consider.

Key Complications that Require Revision Surgery[4]

Not all complications following breast augmentation with implants will necessitate revision surgery, but there are some key reasons why it may be needed or desired. The key issues that could require revision surgery include:

1. Capsular Contraction

All implants form a scar around them, which can shrink, altering the shape and feel of the breast; making them rounder and harder. This is referred to as capsular contraction.

The severity of capsular contracture is rated according to the following system:

➢ Grade 1 is asymptomatic (producing or exhibiting no symptoms). It does not change the size, shape or feel of the breasts.

➢ Grade 2: Usually only mild symptoms are present. Normally, the breasts maintain a consistent shape but feel slightly firmer to the touch.

➢ Grade 3: Symptoms are easily identifiable. The breasts will feel hard to the touch and appear unusually rounded and rigid and nipples often move higher up on the breasts.

➢ Grade 4 produces stiff, deformed breasts. In addition, breasts with grade four capsular contracture usually feel tender and painful.

Treatment of capsular contraction: ThIs previously almost always required invasive surgery but a relatively new non-invasive treatment option is Aspen therapy. This uses ultrasound waves and can be effective for treating stage 2 and 3 capsular contraction.

When this treatment is not effective or in the case of stage 4 capsular contraction a surgical procedure is required to treat. This may be an open or partial capsulotomy which involves surgically removing portions of the scar capsule along with incisions to divide the capsule surrounding the breast implant. The intention is to release the capsule, allowing the implant a greater degree of movement.

Where the capsules are thick or calcified, plastic surgeons will recommend complete removal, referred to as a complete capsulectomy or en-bloc capsulectomy. This procedure is also required if BIA-ALCL or any other type of lymphoma or carcinoma has been diagnosed. The subglandular and subfascial implant placement might need to be changed to a submuscular or dual plane placement, if there is a lack of breast tissue cover following a complete capsulotomy.

2. Sagging

Sagging may be a result of larger implants, pregnancy, breastfeeding or simply gravity and time. Improving the breast shape and position will generally require a breast uplift. Implant replacement may also be recommended at the same time. This is typically done as a single procedure, however, occasionally your surgeon may recommend that re-augmentation is done separately from the uplift procedure.

This can be done in two ways:

➢ Implant removal and an uplift procedure, followed by a second procedure approximately four to six months later, when new implants will be placed.

➢ Implant removal and replacement, followed by an uplift procedure approximately four to six months later.

With modest sagging, that is not an issue, simple implant replacement may be an alternative option to a breast lift. This may involve a larger implant, but, the larger the implant the more likely it will sag over time and a breast uplift may be required at a later date.

3. Implant Malposition

Implants may move sideways, or down if the pocket size is not correct, or when larger, heavier implants are used; particularly in patients with thin tissues. If implants are placed too close then definition of the cleavage may be lost, (symmastia). A double-bubble can arise from a breast implant that sits below the original inframammary crease, where the original crease creates a groove across the lower pole of the breast.

Malposition of the breast implants may require revision surgery. The surgical technique will depend on the direction in which the implants have moved and your tissue and skin elasticity. If the initial position of the implant was subglandular this may need to be changed to a submuscular or dual plane position.

4. Infection, Necrosis and Implant Extrusion

Infection that does not respond to antibiotics could lead to tissue necrosis and implant extrusion. If implants need to be removed due to infection, re-implantation will need to be postponed until the tissues soften, which will normally take many months. If the implant was initially placed in the subglandular position, it may be moved to a submuscular or dual plane position.

5. Breast Implant Associated Anaplastic Large Cell Lymphoma (BIA-ALCL), Breast Implant Associated Squamous Cell Carcinoma (BIA-SCC)

Breast implant associated anaplastic large cell lymphoma (BIA-ALCL) is a rare cancer that is linked to course textured implants.The worldwide withdrawal of Allergan BioCell textured implants in July 2019 was due to the development of breast implant associated anaplastic large cell lymphoma (BIA-ALCL).

The incidence of diagnosis with BIA-ALCL has also been linked to other breast implant manufacturers, however, it is very rare. According to substantial clinical research, the risk associated with BIA-ALCL is presently projected to fall within 0.01% and 0.1%.

Following careful and ongoing evaluation of the current clinical data and the low assessment of risk, this style of Allergan implants are not being recommended for removal by either the:

- UK Medicines and Healthcare products Regulatory Agency (MHRA)
- US Food and Drug Administration (FDA).

All of the official plastic surgery organisations who adhere to a code of ethical behaviour and practice, for the purpose of raising the fundamental requirements for patients safety, have also issued statements regarding the risk of developing BIA-ALCL. In agreement with the MHRA and the FDA each organisation is not recommending removal or replacement of Allergan macro textured implants. The information can be viewed via the links below:

- British Association of Aesthetic Plastic Surgeons (BAAPS)

- British Association of Plastic, Reconstructive and Aesthetic Surgeons (BAPRAS)
- American Society of Plastic Surgery (ASPS)
- Australian Society of Plastic Surgeons (ASPS).

In addition to BIA-ALCL, on September 8, 2022, the US Food and Drug Administration (FDA) published a safety communication that included reports of squamous cell carcinoma (SCC) found in the scar tissue capsule around breast implants.

Such tumours are very rare and have been associated with smooth and textured implant shells, with implants filled with silicone and saline. As of January 15, 2023, the FDA had received 24 medical device reports (MDRs) concerning SCC with breast implants, according to the most recent FDA update, which was released on March 8, 2023.

En bloc capsulectomy (total removal of the implants and scar capsule) is an effective treatment for most people diagnosed with BIA-ALCL or BIA-SCC. People who are not treated quickly enough may require additional treatments, such as chemotherapy, radiotherapy or further surgery.

Breast Implant Removal Surgical Procedures

Choosing to have your breast implants removed can help remove any concerns about the potential of BII or BIA-ALCL that can occur in the capsule that surrounds breast implants. Although it is possible to simply remove implants and the scar capsule, to improve the aesthetic result, a breast uplift procedure may be required.

Autologous fat transfer may be considered where volume is required..

Risks and Complications

As with all surgical procedures the standard risks and complications apply, but because breast implant removal and replacement can require more extensive surgery, certain risks may be higher including:

- Infection
- Seromas, an accumulation of tissue fluid beneath the skin
- Hematomas caused by blood getting trapped beneath the skin
- Death of skin and tissue, referred to as necrosis
- A collapsed lung, often referred to as a pneumothorax (this is extremely rare).

Eight Key Questions to Ask About Breast Implant Revision, Removal or Implant Replacement Surgery

1. Which kind of anaesthetic do you suggest and where will my surgery be performed? (For additional information, see Section One - Regulatory Medical Bodies.)

2. Which surgical approach do you recommend and why?

3. How often have you performed this type of procedure in the past six months?

4. What specific risks and challenges are associated with this surgical technique?

5. What are the most common complications or issues you have encountered with this procedure and how did you resolve them?

6. How do you resolve complications or issues if they arise following the procedure?

7. What type of revision surgery will you offer me if I'm not happy with the result?

8. Is there any charge for additional revision surgery? (Confirmation of the cost and coverage for subsequent revision surgery should be supplied in writing.)

Final Thoughts

There are various reasons for implant removal, or implant removal and replacement. The procedures need to be carefully considered. Treatment may require changing the implant position, mastopexy (uplift) and reshaping of the breast to achieve the best result. Discuss the aesthetic outcome that is most important to you. Ask your plastic surgeon to explain the reasons why they are recommending the incision and surgical technique and the new implants (shell type, filling type, shape and cc volume) if you choose to have an implant replacement procedure.

Your plastic surgeon is the most knowledgeable person to advise you on all of your options and assist you in deciding on the best implants for your specific anatomy and desires. Take your time to make an informed decision.

Annabelle Baugh, Founder of Cosmetic Surgery Advancements

6. EXTRA LARGE BREAST IMPLANTS

Breast augmentation for those seeking extra large breast implants, has gained some popularity over the years. There are various techniques and implants that can be used if you desire extra large implants, which are generally classified as implants with a volume over 800cc.

Extra Large Breast Implant Options

There are four main options if you desire extra large implants over 800cc in volume:

1. **The SILTEX ™ Round BECkER™ 25 Expander/Implants, Cohesive I ™** - This implant has an inner lumen which is filled with 75% saline and an outer lumen which is prefilled with 25% silicone gel. This implant has a total capacity of 1000cc and is made up of two inner lumens, consisting of a 200cc silicone lumen and an 800cc saline lumen.

The saline lumen can be overfilled to 1000cc, making the total implant volume 1200cc, with the silicone outer lumen. However, this will void the warranty. The silicone gel in the outer lumen of the implant makes surface rippling less common, which is a beneficial aspect of this implant.

2. **Saline implants** - The largest saline implants can be filled to 1000cc and some plastic surgeons will overfill to between 1200cc and 2000cc. However, this will void any warranty and increase the potential for rupture.

3. **Custom made silicone filled implants** - There are companies who will custom make silicone implants over 800cc, however, this is an expensive option and you can expect to pay £5000 plus for custom made silicone implants.

4. **Tissue expanders, also known as expandable implants** - These types of implants are filled with saline during the initial procedure. Then saline is added via a port which means they can be expanded while inside your breast. Typically they are expanded to between 1500cc and 2500cc, however some plastic surgeons may be willing to go up to 3000cc or larger. Whilst this type of implant is popular for various reasons in most cases tissue expanders are not meant to be used as long term devices and overfilling them will void any warranty.

Complications and Risks Associated with Large Breast Implants

In addition to the risks and complications associated with breast augmentation surgery with implants, bigger breast implants necessitate a larger implant pocket. This can create issues with tissue support and can increase the risk of:

- Misplacement issues, such as bottoming out, and symmastia (implants meeting in the centre of the chest).
- Infection, necrosis, and implant extrusion
- Nerve injury, which might result in loss of nipple sensation

- Breast tissue atrophy (thinner skin)
- Sagging that could necessitate mastopexy (breast lift) surgery.

Understanding Tissue Expanders for Achieving Extra Large Breast Augmentation

Tissue expanders, often referred to as expandable breast implants, have emerged as an alternative solution to help individuals attain their desired aesthetic goals. Before considering tissue expanders, it's essential to understand exactly how they are utilised if you are seeking extra large breast implants.

The Basics of Tissue Expanders

Tissue expanders are a specialised type of breast implant designed to gradually increase the volume of breast tissue. This may be done in preparation for the insertion of permanent silicone or saline implants, or they may be left in place longer term.

They are particularly useful in cases where individuals desire a more significant size increase beyond what traditional implants can provide. Tissue expanders work by gently stretching the surrounding tissues and skin, enabling the implants to be filled to a greater cc volume than would be possible with just one procedure.

The Process of Using Tissue Expanders

Tissue expanders provide an alternative to having two or more procedures to replace permanent silicone or saline implants, with bigger implants. The process of using tissue expanders for extra large breast augmentation is as follows:

➤ **Initial consultation:** During the initial consultation with your plastic surgeon, your goals and expectations are discussed.

The surgeon will evaluate factors such as your body proportions, skin elasticity, and breast anatomy to determine the suitability of tissue expanders. You may also need to have a second consultation depending on your surgeon, prior to your procedure.

➢ **Insertion of tissue expanders:** In a surgical procedure, a tissue expander is placed in the submuscular position, beneath the chest muscles or in the subglandular position, above the muscle, beneath the breast tissue. This is normally performed under a general anaesthetic but may also be performed under a local anaesthetic. Discuss your options with your surgeon.

If not integral to the expander, an injection port is sited away from the expander, usually in the armpit area, The implant is then partially filled with a sterile saline solution. Tissue expanders can be inserted through any of the standard incisions.

➢ **Gradual expansion:** Over the course of several weeks or months, you will return to the surgeon's office for controlled saline injections, made via the injection port. Following addition of saline you may experience some discomfort, soreness and bruising in your breasts, for around a week.

This gradual expansion process allows the surrounding tissues to stretch and make room for the desired implant cc volume and size. The procedure of filling tissue expanders might take some months, depending on how well your tissues and skin stretch, and the size you want to achieve.

➢ **Replacement with permanent implants:** Once the desired size is achieved, tissue expanders can be replaced with extra large silicone or saline breast implants. You may also decide to keep your tissue expanders in place, but they are not considered to be permanent devices.

Tissue expanders have a thicker outer shell than permanent implants. Replacement of tissue expanders may be recommended if you have noticeable surface rippling or visible implant edges. As silicone implants tend to ripple less and feel more natural than saline, you may prefer to have your tissue expanders exchanged for permanent silicone implants.

Advantages of Tissue Expanders for Extra Large Breast Implants

Tissue expanders may be a solution if you desire implants with a larger cc volume than would be possible to place during an initial breast augmentation, or even a secondary procedure to replace permanent implants.

The key advantages of using tissue expanders for extra large breast augmentation are:

➢ **Reduced number of surgical procedures:** As saline tissue expanders are filled gradually, you can reduce the need to have repeat procedures to replace implants in order to accommodate the cc volume and size implants you want.They can be useful when your surgeon does not believe you will safely be able to accommodate the implant cc volume you want.

➢ **Lower risk of skin/ tissue necrosis (tissue loss) and implant extrusion:** This applies when comparing the use of tissue expanders to large implants, that excessively stretch skin and tissue in one go. The gradual expansion process helps the tissues and skin to adapt more effectively to the larger implants. This means you can accommodate a larger cc volume than you would be able to with just one breast augmentation procedure.

➢ **Customised sizing:** Tissue expanders offer the advantage of gradual size increase and customisation, allowing patients and surgeons to work together to achieve the desired end result.

➢ **Reduced postoperative discomfort:** The incremental expansion approach means the tissue expanders normally leads to reduced postoperative pain, when compared to using a permanent large implant.

➢ **Minimise risk of stretch marks:** Gradual stretching of the skin reduces the likelihood of stretch marks, which can occur when the skin is stretched too quickly. However, stretch marks are still extremely likely if you choose to go significantly bigger than your natural breast size, or want to increase your tissue expanders to over a 1000cc volume.

Risks and Complications of Tissue Expanders

In addition to their advantages in being able to produce large breasts, tissue expanders carry a number of associated risks and complications. Please note these are specific risks that increase when tissue expanders are used instead of permanent implants. All of the normal risks and complications associated with any type of surgical procedure and breast augmentation, also apply when using tissue expanders.

➢ **Increased risk for infection:** Whilst bacterial infections in the tissue surrounding an implants can occur days or weeks following your procedure, implant inflation carries further extra risks. Everytime your skin is punctured there is a potential for infection.

Antibiotics may be prescribed by your surgeon to reduce the risk. If an implant does become infected you may need to go into hospital to have intravenous antibiotics. It may also be necessary to remove the tissue expander. If removed, you may need to wait four to six months for the tissues to settle before you can consider a second surgical procedure to place new implants.

➢ **Increased risk of capsular contraction:** The scar tissue around tissue expanders is more likely to thicken, which can result in capsular contracture. This disorder may result in persistent pain, breast form distortion, and may develop months or even years following your final injection of saline into the expander.

➢ **Increased risk of skin/tissue necrosis (tissue loss) and implant extrusion:** Although stretching the skin and tissue slowly may reduce the risk of necrosis and implant extrusion, expansion will thin the tissues and skin. When overstretching occurs due to the weight of the additional saline this can lead to skin breakdown and implant extrusion. It is important to understand that re-augmentation using implants following the use of tissue expanders is not always possible if skin has become extremely thin.

➤ **Poor aesthetic outcome:** Tissue expanders may produce poor aesthetic outcomes with regards to breast shape and how breasts feel. Saline filled devices do not have the feel of a natural breast. They also have a far higher likelihood of causing skin rippling and, or noticeable implant edges, that can be seen through the skin.

Additional Considerations with Tissue Expanders

Further to the specific risks and complications associated with the use of tissue expanders there are also additional considerations to be aware of, these include;

➤ **Magnetic resonance imaging (MRI) unsafe:** Magnets in valves of tissue expanders may mean they are not safe for MRIs. This could make diagnosis of certain health conditions in the future more complicated.

➤ **Time commitment:** The process of tissue expansion requires time and patience, as it involves multiple visits to the surgeon for saline injections.

➤ **Secondary implant replacement:** Tissue expanders are not considered permanent devices. If you choose to have tissue expanders replaced with permanent implants you will have the potential for complications and risks associated with additional surgery.

➤ **Sagging:** The heavier the implant the more it will sag over time. This could mean you may require a breast uplift procedure later on in life.

➤ **Change of mind:** Extra large breast implants might be

what you desire currently, but this could change as you grow older. Changing tissue expanders for smaller implants later on will typically require a breast lift, and the final result is likely to be compromised, due to thinner skin which is caused by the size of the tissue expanders.

NB: The information provided in this section is related specifically to when tissue expanders are used for aesthetic purposes and not breast reconstruction, which carries its own set of unique complications and risks.

Key Things to Ask About Extra Large Breast Augmentation Surgery

1. How many times have you used this size implant?
2. What are the key complications you have encountered with implants around this size and how did you resolve them?
3. Does this size implant increase the risks and complications and if so which ones and why?

Extra Things to Ask About Tissue Expanders

1. How often have you used tissue expanders for cosmetic purposes in the past three months?
2. What is the maximum cc size you normally will fill tissue expanders?
3. Do you have any concerns that are specifically related to the use of tissue expanders?
4. Have you had any patients develop an infection after having saline injections into a tissue expander?
5. Have you had any cases of extrusion with tissue expanders?
6. How often do you replace tissue expanders for permanent implants?

Final Thoughts

When you want extra large breast implants, tissue expanders may provide a solution that allows for gradual size customisation and a higher cc volume than could be achieved with just one or even two procedures using permanent implants. While the process requires patience and careful planning, the final cc volume can often be far greater than would be possible otherwise.

The alternative may be one or multiple procedures with large permanent implants. If you're considering breast augmentation with extra large implants, take time to consider the increased risks and complications, and the final aesthetic result. Make sure you are prepared for future procedures. These are extremely likely to be required, as tissue expanders are not life time devices and large implants are more likely to sag and change shape over time.

Always consult with a qualified plastic surgeon who is experienced in placing large implants or tissue expander techniques and take on board what they advise you.

Annabelle Baugh, Founder of Cosmetic Surgery Advancements

7. BREAST IMPLANT MANUFACTURERS

When considering breast augmentation or reconstruction surgery with implants, one of the most important decisions is the manufacturer of your breast implants. Almost always plastic surgeons will only use one or two breast implant manufacturers.

Prior to breast augmentation with implants it's critical to ask what breast implant manufacturers you can choose from. Below are eight manufacturers that are popular among plastic surgeons..

Eight Leading Breast Implant Manufacturers

1. Motiva Implants: Motiva is a leading innovator in breast implants. They offer a broad range of implant types, including silicone gel implants and saline implants. Motiva Implants have received the CE Mark and approvals from regulatory bodies worldwide, including the FDA, Health Canada, and TGA in Australia. More information is available on the Motiva implants website.

2. Allergan Aesthetics: Acquired by Actavis, an AbbVie

company. They produce a range of breast implants with silicone and saline fillings. These implants have received the CE Mark in Europe, and have received approval from the FDA and a number of other regulatory agencies around the world. For more information on the types of NATRELLE® Breast Implants, is available in the brochures at <u>Allergan Products</u>.

3. **Sientra:** Known for their "gummy bear" silicone gel implants which have a firm cohesive gel. They produce an extensive range of silicone and saline implants and have received the CE Mark and approval from the FDA and numerous regulatory bodies worldwide. More information and their product catalogue is available on the <u>Sientra website</u>.

4. **Laboratories Arion:** Known for their Monobloc CMC Hydrogel which have obtained the CE Mark and are currently the only implants available as an alternative to silicone filled implants (excluding saline). Hydrogel implants are not available in the UK or the US but are used by plastic surgeons in many other countries throughout Europe. Their range of silicone and saline filled implants are approved by regulatory bodies worldwide. More information and the implant catalogue is available on the <u>Laboratoires Arion website</u>

5. **Mentor:** - Acquired by Johnson & Johnson. They manufacture a range of breast implants with silicone or saline fillings. They have received the CE Mark in Europe, and the FDA and a number of other regulatory organisations throughout the world have granted approval for these implants. For more information about Mentor breast implants please refer to the <u>product section on the Mentor website</u>.

6. **GC Aesthetics:** GC Aesthetics is the parent company of two leading implant manufacturers – Nagor and Eurosilicone. The Nagor facility is in Scotland and England. The Eurosilicone facility is in France. GC Aesthetic breast implants have received the CE Mark in Europe, and approval from the FDA and many more regulatory bodies all over the world.

Their extensive range of breast implants includes three main types: silicone gel implants, saline implants, and innovative structured implants which feature an internal mesh to maintain shape and reduce rippling. For additional information visit the GC Aesthetics website.

7. Sebbin: Their range of silicone gel implants and saline implants have earned the CE Mark in Europe, and approvals from the TGA in Australia. Sebbin implants, which have received the CE Mark, and approval from other regulatory bodies worldwide, including the FDA, Health Canada, and the TGA in Australia. For more information visit the Sebbin website.

8. POLYTECH Health & Aesthetic: Known for their innovative B-lite silicone implant range, which are lighter than conventional silicone implants. Their range includes silicone gel implants and saline implants and they have earned the CE Mark in Europe, and approvals from regulatory bodies worldwide, including the TGA in Australia visit the POLYTECH website.

Breast Implant Warranties

All breast implants will come with a warranty and you can ask to look at this prior to your breast augmentation. Check how long the warranty covers the implants for and what surgical costs are covered in the case of ruptured or withdrawn implants.

Complications Associated with Breast Implants: Know the Options if Issues Arise

Unfortunately, implants can rupture over time or cause complications like capsular contraction. This may require replacement or removal.

Be prepared to discuss:

- Uplift, reshaping or altering implant placement

- Switching implant size, texture or profile
- Mastopexy techniques if uplift is needed.

Breast Implant Withdrawals

In the past decade, some types of breast implants have been withdrawn from the market, including:

➢ **Lipomatrix Inc Trilucent Breast Implants**

These implants are filled with soya bean oil and were withdrawn in the UK and Europe in 2000 (FDA approval was not granted for use in the US)

An independent study was conducted to evaluate the potential dangers associated with the soya bean oil filling. It was discovered that there is a possibility of exposure to toxic breakdown products that can react with tissue surrounding the implant. As a result, the <u>MHRA advice is to remove Trilucent breast implants</u>. The study, however, found no indication that Trilucent breast implants caused risks to health, and it appears that removing the implants eliminates any possible risks.

➢ **Poly Implant Prothese (PIP) and NovaGoldTM: Hydrogel Breast Implants**

There were two manufacturers of hydrogel-filled breast implants that were available in the UK. Both were withdrawn in the UK and Europe in 2000 (FDA approval was not granted for use in the US).

The study conducted by the Medical Devices Agency (MDA) uncovered shortcomings in the manufacturers biological safety studies and concluded that there was insufficient evidence to thoroughly analyse either filler material. There has been no definitive risk found and there is no indication that they can cause harm or that they should be removed from women who already have these implants. The issue is only with how the safety of the hydrogel fillers has been evaluated.

➢ **Poly Implant Prothese (PIP) Silicone Breast Implants**

These implants were withdrawn in the UK and Europe in 2010 (FDA approval was not granted for use in the US).

The French medical device regulatory body (AFSSAPS) told the MHRA that they had recalled and suspended the marketing, distribution, export, and usage of PIP silicone gel filled breast implants. Immediately following this, the MHRA advised UK doctors to discontinue use PIP implants.

The compromised implants were examined for genotoxicity (the risk of cancer), chemical toxicity of the filler material, and mechanical characteristics of the implant shell by AFSSAPS. The AFSSAPS mechanical examination of the implant shells indicates that they are more prone to rupture. The French Ministry of Health recommended that all women with PIP implants have them removed in December 2011.

According to tests by the Australian government's Therapeutic Goods Administration (TGA), PIP silicone gel filled breast implants met all of the relevant international requirements for this type of product, including those for gel cytotoxicity and shell strength. The MHRA found no evidence of genotoxicity or chemical toxicity in the filler material, and does not suggest routine removal of PIP silicone gel breast implants in the UK.

More information is available in the Poly Implant Prothèse (PIP) Review prepared by the UK Department of Health

➢ **Allergan Breast Implants**

Allergan voluntarily issued a worldwide withdrawal of the below brands of breast implants, following a request from the FDA in July 2019. This was due to an association with Breast Implant Associated Anaplastic Large Cell Lymphoma (BIA-ALCL), a rare type of lymphoma linked to textured implants.

Brand	Style
Natrelle Saline	168, 363, 468
Natrelle and McGhan 410 and 410 Soft Touch	LL, LM, LF, LX, ML, MM, MF, MX, FL, FM, FF, FX
Natrelle 510 Dual-Gel	LX, MX, FX
Natrelle INSPIRA	TRL, TRLP, TRM, TRF, TRX, TSL, TSLP, TSM, TSF, TSX, TCL, TCLP, TCM, TCF, TCX
Natrelle and McGhan Round Gel	110, 110 Soft Touch, 120, 120 Soft Touch
Natrelle Komuro	KML, KMM, KLL, and KLM
Natrelle Ritz Princess	RML, RMM, RFL, RFM
Natrelle 150 double lumen implants	Full Height and Short Height
Natrelle 133 tissue expanders with and without suture tabs	133FV, 133MV, 133LV, 133MX, 133SX, 133SV,
Natrelle 133 Plus tissue expander styles with and without suture tabs	133P-FV, 133P-MV, 133P-LV, 133P-MX, 133P-SX, 133P-SV

Source: FDA

Regulators worldwide do not currently recommend removal or replacement of any of the withdrawn Allergan implant brands when there are no signs or symptoms of BIA-'ALCL. Ask your surgeon about monitoring for BIA-ALCL and how you can get a diagnosis if you experience any concerning symptoms.

Final Thoughts

This demonstrates the importance of selecting your breast implant manufacturer carefully and working with a plastic surgeon you can trust. Always ensure you are provided with the manufacturer's patent implant card and warranty information for future reference.

Annabelle Baugh, Founder of Cosmetic Surgery Advancements

C. BREAST UPLIFT AND REDUCTION SURGERY

1. BREAST UPLIFT WITH OR WITHOUT IMPLANTS

In the world of cosmetic breast surgery a breast lift, medically known as a mastopexy, can be a game changer. It's a surgical procedure that can transform the appearance of sagging breasts – even if you already have breast implants. Moreover, a breast lift can be combined with the addition of breast implants to create more volume if desired.

There are multiple aspects to a breast lift, each with its unique approach. The type of lift that suits you best depends on a number of factors:

- Degree of uplift you're aiming for
- Extent of skin removal needed
- What scarring you're prepared to accept.

A breast lift is not about increasing the size of your breasts, although, if you choose to have a breast lift with implants you can opt to increase your breast volume. In this section we cover all of the essential information you need about a breast lift as a solo procedure, a breast lift with existing implants and combining a breast lift with implants.

Types of Breast Lift Surgery

There are four key techniques used when performing a breast lift procedure. The type of breast lift you decide to have will be based on the end aesthetic result you want to achieve and your current anatomy. Each technique has its own distinct benefits and disadvantages that you should consider in order to make an informed decision.

Ultimately the amount of droop you have will influence the technique required and your plastic surgeon will be able to advise why they recommend a specific type of breast lift, your options and how the technique used will create the closest possible result, to the one you desire.

1. Crescent Breast Lift (Scarless Lift)

The crescent breast lift is sometimes referred to as the scar free breast lift, however, this is not accurate. As with all techniques the crescent breast lift requires incisions and will therefore create scars. The key difference is this type of breast lift is minimally invasive and only requires an incision around the upper half of the areola.

➢ **A desire for minimal scarring:** Out of all types of breast lifts, the crescent breast lift requires the smallest incision, but gives the smallest correction. Due to the location of the scar, in most cases it will fade and become almost undetectable. However, it's important to understand that the quality of the scar will depend on how you heal, and might be clearly visible if it does not heal well.

➢ **Mild sagging:** This procedure is only suitable for individuals who are contending with a mild degree of breast ptosis. Should the sagging be severe, alternative types of breast lifts might be more suitable.

➢ **Small to medium breast size:** The crescent lift is more effective for females with less voluminous breasts, generally between a B to C bra cup size. This is attributed to the fact that smaller breasts typically necessitate less lifting and reshaping, rendering this minimally invasive procedure possible.

➤ **Preference for Subtle Results:** The crescent lift procedure is capable of elevating the nipple by an approximate two centimetres. If your preference leans towards a subtle change rather than a dramatic transformation, this breast lift procedure could be the most suitable to achieve your desired results.

2. Periareolar Breast Lift (Donut Lift)

Alternatively, known as the doughnut lift, the periareolar lift is suitable for mild to moderate sagging. Stepping up from the crescent lift, this procedure is more common as it allows for additional skin removal, reshaping of existing breast tissue and relocation of the nipple.

➤ **Scarring:** A ring of skin, forming a doughnut shape, is removed to allow the nipple to be positioned at a higher level. The incisions are then sewn together, leaving a scar at the outer edge of the areola. Although scars may be noticeable, depending on how well they heal, typically, the resultant scar blends well with the surrounding skin and is well hidden.

➤ **Moderate sagging:** This method can address breasts with moderate sagging and excess skin. Where increased volume is required, it can also be combined with breast implants.

➤ **Medium breast size:** The periareolar lift is most suitable for small to medium sized breasts.

➤ **Require moderate lift:** The periareolar lift is capable of relocating the nipple and creating a moderate degree of lift. If your objective is for a modest change in shape and degree of sagging, rather than a substantial transformation, this type of breast lift could be the ideal solution to achieve your desired outcome.

3. Vertical Breast Lift (Lollipop Lift)

The lollipop lift, also known as the vertical breast lift, is well suited for moderate to more severe sagging. With this technique there is also greater access to reshape the existing breast tissue.

➢ **Scarring:** This technique requires an incision around the areola and another vertical one, running from the middle of the bottom edge of the areola to the breast crease, resulting in a lollipop-shaped scar.

➢ **Medium to large breasts:** Ideally suited for individuals with medium to larger sized breasts.

➢ **Moderate to severe sagging:** The vertical scar lift repositions the nipple and allows reshaping to give a substantial correction.

4. Inverted T or Anchor Breast Lift

The inverted T lift, also known as the anchor lift, is used for large breasts with significant sagging and excess skin. This technique allows skin excision in the vertical plane and the most visibility to reshape breast tissue.

➢ **Scarring:** The anchor lift requires three incisions, one around the areola, a second one vertically, and a third along the crease of the breast. This will create an inverted T or anchor shaped scar on the breast. Whilst scars are more visible they should sit in the bra area.

➢ **Large breasts:** This might be the best breast lift option for large breasts with significant sagging.

➢ **Severe sagging:** If you're looking for a significant uplift and change in breast shape this technique allows for the greatest removal of excess skin.

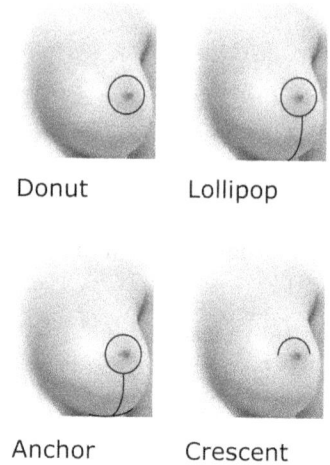

Breast uplift scar locations

Breast Lift with Pre-Existing Breast Implants

It is possible to have a breast lift with pre-existing breast implants. The breast lift will simply remove excess skin and lift the nipples to correct sagging, and improve the overall shape of the breasts.

Depending on the age of your implants and the thickness of the capsule that surrounds them, it may be necessary to exchange your implants at the same time. Your plastic surgeon will be able to advise you of the best course of action.

Combining Breast Implants with a Breast Lift

All types of breast lift procedures can be combined with breast implants if there is a desire to increase the volume of the breasts. This can be done as a single operation or split into two stages. The extent of your sagging and the quality of your tissues will determine which is best for you. One stage surgery is more complex and not advocated by all surgeons.

- **One Stage Surgical Procedure**

When a breast lift is combined with a breast implant in one procedure a phenomenal change in the position and shape of the breasts is possible.

Breast lift procedures that are combined with implants tend to be most suitable for small to moderate sized breasts, particularly when volume has been lost. Below are a few of the key considerations.

➤ **Implant placement:** The position of implants is determined by the quality and thickness of the breast tissue. If thin, they will be placed under the pectoralis muscle in the upper pole.

➤ **Type of Implants:** Silicone gel implants are generally recommended over saline implants, as they tend to look and feel more natural and are less prone to rippling. Implants are available in various shapes, widths, heights and projections, for more information please refer to - Breast Augmentation With Breast Implants

➤ **Risks and complications:** Placement of breast implants during a breast lift may increase the risk of complications. These will be discussed by your surgeon in deciding which procedure is best for you.

➤ **Recovery time:** While individuals may normally resume light activities within a week, engaging in more strenuous exercises and lifting heavy objects should be avoided for at least six weeks to facilitate optimal healing. Post surgery, patients will experience some swelling, bruising, and discomfort, which will gradually diminish over four to six weeks. Adhering to the surgeon's postoperative care instructions, including wearing support garments, is crucial during the recovery phase.

➤ **Time Until Results:** The final results of a breast lift become more apparent as the healing progresses. Although some initial changes are noticeable shortly after the procedure, skin stretches to its natural tension, the breasts settle into their new position over the course of around three to six months.

The final results will also depend on the type of procedure, surgical technique and placement of breast implants. It is essential to maintain regular follow-up appointments with the surgeon to monitor progress and address any concerns throughout the recovery process.

➢ **Long term complications:** When implants are placed during the breast lift procedure there is an increased potential for implant misplacement and future sagging, referred to as bottoming out.

- **Two Stage Surgical Procedure**

When breast implants are desired with a breast lift, it may be best approached as a two-stage operation to optimise long-term outcomes and minimise potential complications. This will be discussed by your surgeon.

In the initial stage, the plastic surgeon concentrates on lifting and reshaping the breasts to establish a suitable size and shape that will accommodate the subsequent implants. Delaying the placement of implants for a period between six to nine months is generally recommended, before proceeding to the second stage to insert breast implants. This is to allow the scars to mature and soften. Performing surgery in two stages reduces the risk of wound healing problems creating issues and, for some surgeons, better shaping and more accurate implant positioning

A consideration that may influence the recommendation for a two-stage procedure is the possibility of achieving satisfactory results from the initial breast lift surgery, without breast implants. The two-stage procedure can provide flexibility and allows for treatment options, based on the way an individual heals following a breast lift, and their desired results.

➤ **Implant Placement:** The position of implants is determined by the quality and thickness of the breast tissue. If thin, they will be placed under the pectoralis muscle in the upper pole.

➤ **Type of Implants:** Silicone gel implants are generally recommended over saline implants, as they tend to look and feel more natural and are less prone to rippling. Implants are available in various shapes, widths, heights and projections, for more information please refer to - Breast Augmentation With Breast Implants

➤ **Risks and Complications:** Performing a breast lift as a two stage procedure carries the risks of another surgery. It can minimise the risk of wound healing problems creating issues for the implant. Some surgeons find reshaping the breast easier without an implant and choose to carry out augmentation once the new breast shape is established.

➤ **Recovery Time:** While light activities may resume within a week, avoiding strenuous exercises and heavy lifting for at least six weeks is crucial for optimal healing. Patients will experience temporary swelling, bruising, and discomfort, gradually diminishing over four to six weeks.

Following all of the surgeon's postoperative care instructions, including wearing support garments, is imperative during the recovery phase.

➤ **Final Results:** The final results of a breast lift become increasingly evident as the healing progresses. While some initial changes may be noticeable shortly after the procedure, the breasts settle into their new position over approximately three to six months. The ultimate outcome following the second procedure is influenced by the procedure type, surgical technique, and implant placement. Regular follow-up appointments with the surgeon are essential to monitor progress and detect any potential problems throughout the recovery process.

➢ **Long-Term Complications:** Although the potential for some complications may be reduced with a two stage procedure, the inclusion of implants following a breast lift still raises the potential for complications such as implant misplacement and future sagging, known as bottoming out.

Breast Lift Risks and Complications

A breast lift procedure is a significant decision, and while the benefits are often transformative, it is crucial to be well informed about potential risks and complications. This list provides a comprehensive overview of the potential challenges associated with breast lift surgery.

➢ **Anaesthesia:** Typically breast lifts are performed under general anaesthetic, although the crescent and periareolar lift may sometimes be performed under local anaesthetic. For more information about the risks of general anaesthetic and complications associated with all types of surgery please refer to Section Two, a. <u>Anaesthetic and Surgery Risks and Complications</u>

➢ **Bleeding:** Although uncommon, bleeding can occur either immediately or after surgery. An additional operation may be necessary to drain any collection. Rarely blood transfusion may be required. Pre-surgery discussions should include medications and the management of high blood pressure.

➢ **Swelling, bruising, and pain:** Following the surgery, anticipate breast swelling and bruising, which typically subside over the course of several weeks. Long-term pain is infrequent. Ibuprofen or other simple analgesic agents are usually all that is requires

➢ **Seroma:** An accumulation of fluid in the breast may require drainage through the skin or an additional operation, potentially affecting the success of the surgery.

➢ **Hematoma:** A build-up of blood in the breast could necessitate draining or a second procedure, which could compromise the surgical outcome.

➤ **Infection:** Wound infections might necessitate antibiotics or further surgery. This can impact on the overall outcome of the procedure and the recovery time. It is important to inform the surgeon of any nipple discharge before surgery to effectively address infection risks.

➤ **Healing problems:** Issues such as wound edge separation may arise, requiring dressing changes or additional surgery. Smokers face increased risks and smoking should be stopped in advance of surgery.

➤ **Loss of blood supply:** Tissue loss (necrosis) from problems with the blood supply, can affect skin, fat and the nipple. This may necessitate another operation, and can result in lumpiness or distortion of the breast. If affected, nipple reconstruction may be required.

➤ **Sensation changes:** Altered sensation, numbness near the scars, and of the nipple can occur. These may be permanent.

➤ **Asymmetry:** Breasts may not achieve symmetry. Any irregularities may improve with time or require a minor corrective procedure.

➤ **Scars:** The quality of scarring is down to how you heal. Scars may be broad, thickened, and, sometimes, painful. This may necessitate corrective surgical intervention.

➤ **Breast implant problems:** In cases where breast implants are inserted during or after a breast lift, there is a potential for breast implant extrusion to occur as a result of an infection or a breakdown in wound healing. There are several other complications associated with breast implants, for more information please refer to - Breast Augmentation Surgery

Eight Questions to Ask About Breast Uplift Procedures[5]

1. Which anaesthetic do you recommend and where is my procedure going to be performed? (See Section One, Regulatory Medical Bodies, for further details.)

2. Which surgical technique would you suggest, and why?

3. In the past six months, how many times have you carried out this kind of surgery?

4. What particular potential risks and challenges correspond to this surgical method?

5. Which are the most frequent problems or complications you have had with this type of procedure, and how did you address them?

6. If problems or complications come up after the procedure has been performed, how do you handle them?

7. In the event that I'm unhappy with the outcome, what kind of corrective surgery will you provide?

8. Are additional revision surgeries charged for? (A written confirmation of the price and reimbursement for any further revision procedures that are provided should be issued.)

Final Thoughts

A breast lift can enhance both your appearance and confidence. If you are unhappy with the shape of your breasts you may prefer to have a breast lift to other options such as implants or autologous fat transfer, or combining these options with a breast lift might be necessary to achieve the aesthetic outcomes you are hoping for. Informed decisions about the type of breast lift procedure and if desired, combining a breast lift with breast implants, need to be based on your own unique concerns and should always be made in consultation with a qualified plastic surgeon experienced with breast lifts.

Annabelle Baugh, Founder of Cosmetic Surgery Advancements

2. BREAST REDUCTION SURGERY

Breast reduction surgery, also known as reduction mammoplasty, involves the removal of excess breast tissue, fat, and skin to achieve a more proportionate and comfortable breast size. The procedure is designed to improve the aesthetic look of breasts by addressing sagging, improving overall breast shape and often adjusting nipple position as well as reducing size. By reducing the weight of the breasts, physical discomfort associated with large breasts is normally alleviated.

In this article, we will delve into the surgical techniques, recovery times, potential risks, and the long term results that may be a result from breast reduction surgery.

Liposuction Breast Reduction (LBR)

Liposuction assisted breast reduction is sometimes referred to as scarless breast reduction. The technique is not employed often as it is best suited to patients with fatty breast tissue, good skin elasticity and minimal sagging.

➢ **Technique:** Tumescent liposuction is the preferred technique and the procedure can be performed under local anaesthetic or general anaesthetic.

➢ **Recovery time:** Dressing will need changing in the first 72 hours following the procedure and, typically, most patients return to work and daily activities within three to five days. Low impact exercise can be safely initiated after two weeks, provided proper support is maintained.

More intense aerobic exercise and weight lifting should be avoided for 6 weeks. Throughout the six month healing period, it is crucial for to consistently wear appropriate support to optimise elastic tissue recoil and achieve maximal correction of sagging and the degree of ptosis once the breast tissue is healed.

➢ **Complications and risks:** The primary complication associated with LBR are haematomas, which may need drains and additional treatment to resolve. Similar to standard liposuction cases, infection is a rare occurrence. If redness indicative of infection appears, oral antibiotics are recommended.

In cases where an infection progresses, despite oral antibiotics, intravenous antibiotic medication may need to be administered in hospital. Vigilance and adherence to postoperative care guidelines contribute to a smoother recovery process for patients undergoing LBR.

➢ **Scars:** The incisions made for tumescent liposuction are very small typically just 1 to 2 cm in width and once healed are very difficult to detect, hence the name the scarless breast reduction.

➢ **Final results:** This technique will reduce breast size and sagging but will not reposition nipples that are low down, although a slight degree of lift may be achieved. Depending on breast size, LBR may offer a long term solution, however, for reduction of larger breasts, this technique is unlikely to produce an optimal breast shape or nipple location.

Traditional Breast Reduction Surgical Techniques

There are three surgical techniques that are generally recommended for optimal breast reduction results. Prior to choosing a surgical technique, with the support of a plastic surgeon during a consultation, it can be helpful to consider to what degree the shape, nipple location and overall appearance of your breasts is important to you, vs the reduction in physical discomfort from large breasts.

Of course the ideal breast reduction procedure will address physical discomfort by reducing breast size and weight, while producing an aesthetically pleasing breast shape and nipple location. With larger breasts that require a more significant amount of glandular and fatty tissue to be removed, and or, with significant sagging and low nipples, a compromise may need to be reached if you have a desire for limited scarring.

1. Periareolar Breast Reduction

Generally the periareolar breast reduction is not recommended for women who desire a reduction of more than one bra cup or with severe ptosis.

➤ **Technique:** This technique required two incisions one around the edge of the areola and then another one a little further out from the edge of the areola. This creates a donut shape and allows for removal of excess skin and breast tissue. The skin is then sutured to the edge of the areola.

➤ **Scars:** Scars will be located around the areola and once healed should be very discreet. Occasionally puckering and creasing around the scar may occur which can impact the overall shape of the areola and breasts.

2. Vertical or "Lollipop" Breast Reduction

Normally recommended for women with moderate sagging, the vertical or lollipop technique is most appropriate for women seeking a reduction of breast size around two bra cups.

➤ **Technique:** The vertical or "lollipop" breast reduction technique involves a circular incision around the areola and a vertical incision down to the centre of the breast crease. Due to increased access to breast tissue, this technique often results in a more pleasing breast shape.

➤ **Scars:** The scar resembles a lollipop, hence the nickname lollipop reduction. However, although the horizontal scar down the bottom section of the breast is more noticeable, this scar should fade and become a lot less apparent over time.

3. Anchor Breast Reduction

The anchor breast reduction is the most common breast reduction surgical technique which allows for substantial reshaping of the breast tissue and relocation of the nipple. This technique can be used to reduce breast size by two or more bra sizes and significantly reduces sagging.

➤ **Technique:** It involves making an anchor shaped incision around the areola, extending vertically down the breast and horizontally along the breast crease. Excess breast tissue, fat, and skin are removed, and the remaining tissue is reshaped to achieve a more proportional and aesthetically pleasing result.

➤ **Scars:** The anchor technique employs an additional incision to the vertical breast reduction. This incision is made along the crease of the beasts, but once healed the scar is generally well hidden. For this reason this technique tends to be preferred as it allows better access and for greater reshaping of breast tissue, often resulting in an improved breast shape.

Breast Reduction Recovery Times

Recovery times will differ depending on the technique employed. Below is a general guideline of what to expect following a traditional surgical breast reduction.

Immediate Post-Surgery:

Swelling, bruising, and discomfort which is normally controlled by painkillers for the first three to five days. A surgical bra must be worn to support the breasts.

DURING THE FIRST TWO WEEKS:

- Rest and limited arm movement are recommended
- Pain medication is often prescribed to manage discomfort
- A follow up appointment is typically arranged approximately 10 days following the procedure to monitor healing.

DURING THE FIRST **four to six weeks:**

- Most patients can return to non-strenuous activities, but vigorous exercise and heavy lifting should be avoided
- Swelling begins to subside, and breasts shape should improve
- Incisions should heal, absorbable sutures are often used, but another follow up appointment during this period may be required if sutures need to be removed.

SIX WEEKS TO SIX MONTHS:

- Full recovery time varies, but most patients can resume normal activities after six to 12 weeks
- Breast shape will continue to improve
- Scars continue to fade over time.

SIX TO TWELVE MONTHS:

- The final breast shape will typically be apparent by this point
- Underwired bras can normally be worn
- Swelling should have completely subsided
- Scars should have faded and become significantly flatter and finer.

Risks and Complications of Breast Reduction Surgery

Making the choice to have breast reduction surgery performed is a big one, and although the results can be significant, it's important to know about the associated risks and complications. The potential problems associated with breast reduction surgery are fully outlined in the list that follows:

- **Anaesthesia:** Breast lifts are typically performed under general anaesthesia, although certain occasionally they may be performed using local anaesthesia. Refer to Section Two, a. <u>Anaesthetic and Surgery Risks and Complications</u>, for more information on the risks associated with general anaesthesia and surgery.

- **Bleeding:** Bleeding may happen during or right after surgery, necessitating further surgery to get rid of any hematoma (accumulated blood). Rarely, a blood transfusion might be required. Pre-operative counselling will ask about prescription drugs for control of high blood pressure and blood thinners.
- **Swelling, bruising, and pain:** Post-surgery, expect breast swelling and bruising, which normally diminish over the first two to three weeks. Long term pain is infrequent, and simple analgesic agents like ibuprofen are usually sufficient.
- **Seroma:** An excessive buildup of fluid in the breast could necessitate a second procedure or drains, which might affect the outcome of what was originally done.
- **Infection:** Infections in the wounds may necessitate antibiotics or additional surgery, which will impact the final result and length of recuperation. It is important to notify the surgeon of any discharge from the nipple prior to surgery in order to minimise the risk of infection.
- **Delayed healing:** There's a chance that wound edge separation will happen, requiring more surgery or dressing changes. It is important to stop smoking before surgery because smokers have a higher risk of this occurring.
- **Loss of blood supply:** Issues with blood supply may lead to tissue loss (necrosis) affecting skin, fat, and the nipple. This may require another operation and can result in lumpiness or distortion of the breast, potentially necessitating nipple reconstruction.
- **Sensation Changes:** Changes in feeling, including numbness around the scar and in the nipple, could happen and might even be permanent.

- **Asymmetry:** Achieving symmetry may be challenging, and any irregularities may improve with time or require minor corrective procedures.
- **Scars:** Individual healing determines the quality of scarring. Large, thickened, and occasionally painful scars may require corrective surgery to address. The use of Solution for Scars, before surgery and until the scars mature can help.

Eight Questions to Ask About Breast Reduction Procedure

1. What is your recommended anaesthesia and where will my procedure be carried out? (For further information, read Section One, Regulatory Medical Bodies.)

2. What is your recommended surgical method and why?

3. In the previous six months, how many times did you do this kind of procedure?

4. What specific risk factors and difficulties come with using this surgical technique?

5. How do you resolve the issues or complications you had with this procedure?

6. After the treatment, how do you handle any problems or complications that may arise?

7. If I'm unhappy with the outcome, what kind of revision surgery do you offer?

8. Does extra revision surgery have an expense attached? (In written form, the cost and exact cover for any further revision surgery should be confirmed.)

Final Thoughts

Breast reduction surgery is a transformative procedure that goes beyond aesthetic enhancements, also, providing significant physical benefits. While the decision to undergo surgery should be carefully considered, the long term results are often life changing for those who choose this path. As with any surgical procedure, it is crucial to consult with a plastic surgeon to discuss individual goals, expectations, and potential risks.

Annabelle Baugh, Founder of Cosmetic Surgery Advancements

D. COSMETIC NIPPLE SURGERY

1. AREOLA REDUCTION SURGERY

The areola, the pigmented area surrounding the nipple, plays a crucial role in defining the overall appearance of the breast. Areola reduction surgery is a cosmetic procedure designed to alter the size and shape of the areolas to achieve a more balanced and proportionate look. This section covers all of the details you should know about the procedure, recovery and risks and complications.

The Procedure

➤ **Anaesthetic:** Areola reduction surgery is typically performed under local anaesthesia on an outpatient basis, Twilight sedation may be administered to aid patient comfort if desired.

➤ **Technique:** Removal of excess areolar tissue creates a more proportionate and symmetrical appearance. To correct mild sagging periareolar breast reduction requires two incisions, one around the areola's margin and the other a little bit farther out. This produces a donut-like shape and makes it possible to remove extra breast tissue and skin. After that, the skin is sutured around the border of the areola.

➤ **Scars:** The surgeon strategically places incisions along the natural border of the areola to minimise visible scarring. The incisions are closed using fine dissolvable stitches. This careful approach allows for precise removal of excess tissue while maintaining the integrity of the surrounding skin.

After they heal, the scars that surround the areola should be inconspicuous. The result is determined by how you heal. When mild sagging has been corrected with the periareolar breast reduction technique, there is a risk that the form of the areola and breasts may be affected by puckering and creasing around the scar.

➤ **Recovery time:** After surgery, dressings will need to be changed for the first 72 hours. Recovery from areola reduction surgery is generally swift, with most patients able to return to their daily activities within a three to five days. After two weeks, low-impact exercise can be started safely as long as the right kind of support is worn. It's recommended to refrain from heavier weights and more strenuous aerobic training for six weeks.

➤ **Final results:** After six weeks the majority of the swelling will normally have subsided and the final results should be more apparent. The final outcome may take up to six months to be fully visible .

Complications and Risks of: Areola Reduction Surgery

Like any surgical procedure, it's important to note that individual experiences may vary, and not everyone will encounter these issues. Before undergoing any surgery, individuals should thoroughly discuss potential risks and complications with their plastic surgeon. Here is a list of possible complications and risks associated with areola reduction surgery:

- **Infection:** Any surgical procedure carries a risk of infection, which may occur at the incision site.

- **Bleeding:** Excessive bleeding during or after the surgery is a potential risk.
- **Changes in Sensation:** Some individuals may experience changes in nipple or breast sensation, including increased or decreased sensitivity.
- **Nipple Necrosis:** Factors such as poor blood circulation or individual healing responses may contribute to slow or incomplete wound healing. In rare cases, reduced blood supply to the nipple can lead to tissue death, resulting in nipple necrosis.
- **Difficulty Breastfeeding:** Areola reduction surgery should not impact breastfeeding, as it does not damage the milk ducts or alter nipple function.
- **Asymmetry:** Achieving perfect symmetry can be challenging, and there is a risk of uneven results between the two breasts.
- **Undercorrection or Overcorrection:** The surgeon may undercorrect or overcorrect the size of the areola, leading to unsatisfactory results.
- **Pigmentation Changes:** The areola's colour may change, and pigmentation irregularities may occur as a result of the surgery.
- **Scarring:** Scarring is a common outcome of surgery, and the extent of scarring can vary among individuals. In some cases, the scars may be more noticeable or take longer to fade. There is also a risk of developing scar tissue around the areola, causing it to become firm or distorted.

Seven Key Questions to Ask About Areola Reduction Surgery

1. Which kind of anaesthesia do you provide, and where will my surgery be performed? (For further information, see Section One - Regulatory Medical Bodies.)

2. How many times have you done this procedure in the past six months?

3. Which surgical complications or issues have you encountered most frequently, and how did you resolve them?

4. Have any patients had nipple loss or necrosis?

5. In the event that issues or complications arise following surgery, how do you address them?

6. What type of corrective surgery will you provide if I'm not satisfied with the result?

7. Are further revision operations subject to fees? (Confirmation of payments and precise payment of all medical expenses should be provided in writing.)

Final Thoughts

Areola reduction surgery is a relatively minor surgical procedure, but the potential for unsatisfactory results should be carefully considered before deciding to go ahead. As with any type of cosmetic surgery if you are unhappy with the appearance of your areolas it can be very worthwhile. It's essential to speak with a plastic surgeon about personal objectives, expectations, and possible complications before choosing to go ahead.

Annabelle Baugh, Founder of Cosmetic Surgery Advancements

2. INVERTED NIPPLE CORRECTION

Treatment aims to address nipples that retract or invert into the breast rather than protruding outward; caused by short lactiferous, (breast), ducts. As a first line treatment, use the Niplette, designed to stretch the short ducts, with prolonged stretching over a number of weeks. Projection will be maintained by the muscle within the nipple and can be helped by wearing nipple bars, fixed through a piercing.

When non-surgical treatments are unsuccessful, surgery can be considered, but stretching the ducts can avoid the need to divide them; damaging breast function.

The specific surgical technique and incisions used vary based on the severity of the inversion, the underlying anatomical factors, and the preferences of the patient and the plastic surgeon.

Typically, outpatient inverted nipple correction surgery is done under local anaesthesia, though patients may request twilight sedation if they would like to feel more at ease. The procedure generally takes between 20 and 30 minutes.

Surgery will leave scars around the base of the nipple, with scars on the areola if a sling technique is used to hold the nipple out. Tight lactiferous ducts will require division, to allow the nipple to project. Use of the Niplette can avoid this damage to breast function and increase the success rate of surgery, if required. With very tight ducts a spacer may be placed after division to reduce the risk of recurrent inversion.

Recovery Time and Final Results

The recovery period for inverted nipple surgery is generally brief. Most patients can start undertaking light activities within 24 to 48 hours. Avoid pressure on the nipple by cutting the end out of an old bra, or wear a feeding bra. Mild swelling and bruising is common but these symptoms typically resolve within a week. Strenuous lifting or exertion should be avoided for two weeks and nipple protection may be required for between 4 and six weeks.

It may take several weeks or months for the final projection and shape to be apparent and nipples may appear slightly wider or have a different texture initially. Nipple sensation can be affected temporarily. Once healed sensation should be generally unaffected and the nipple should retain the ability to contract.Over the course of a year, the majority of nipples will lose about 50% of their initial postprocedure projection.

Complications and Risks of: Inverted Nipple Reduction Surgery

- Hematomas (collection of blood under the skin)
- Seromas (collection of fluid under the skin)
- Infection and the need for antibiotics or additional procedures
- Delayed wound healing
- Wound dehiscence (reopening of wound)

- Partial or total loss of nipple/areola due to necrosis (death of tissue)
- Nipple asymmetry or areola irregularity
- Nerve damage causing numbness or decreased sensation in nipples and, or breast
- Difficulty breastfeeding due to nipple/duct damage.

Seven Key Questions to Ask About Inverted Nipple Surgery

1. Which anaesthetic type do you offer, and in what facility will my surgery take place? (See Section One - Regulatory Medical Bodies for more details.)

2. In the last six months, how many times have you carried out this surgery?

3. Which are the most frequent problems or complications you have had with this surgery, and how did you solve them?

4. Have any patients suffered with necrosis or nipple loss?

5. If problems or complications come up after the surgical procedure, how do you handle them?

6. In the event that I'm unhappy with the outcome, what kind of corrective surgery will you offer?

7. Are additional revision surgeries charged for? (Verification of fees and exact coverage of all hospital costs should be provided in writing.)

Final Thoughts

It's essential to consult with a plastic surgeon to determine the severity of the inversion, the elasticity of the tissues, and the desired outcome to recommend the most effective approach for achieving a natural looking and lasting correction.

Annabelle Baugh, Founder of Cosmetic Surgery Advancements

E. BREAST SURGERY SCAR TREATMENTS

Undergoing breast surgery is a significant and often life changing experience. While the results can be transformative, the resulting scars may impact your satisfaction with the results of your surgery. Fortunately, advancements in medical science and skincare have led to various effective treatments for minimising and managing breast surgery scars.

In this section, we'll explore a range of scar treatment options to help you make informed decisions on your scar care journey, for the best possible outcome regardless of your chosen surgical procedure.

Types of Surgical Scars

Cosmetic breast surgery scars will hopefully heal to be fine white lines and will not cause any issues. Scars may not settle as expected, due to complications, such as an infection, or simply due to the way an individual heals. Scars that may require scar treatments following surgery include:

➢ **Keloid scars:** These scars are typically a darker colour, raised, smooth, and firm; They grow larger than the initial inci sion, invading the skin around, and may also cause discomfort in the affected area. If scar treatment is not received, they usually do not fade or flatten.

➤ **Hypertrophic scars:** These scars are usually elevated and stiff, but do not grow to be larger than the initial incision. The scars area may be uncomfortable or difficult to move. However, they will normally fade and flatten over time.

➤ **Linear scars:** These scars might be thick, whiter or darker than the surrounding skin, red and lumpy, or any combination of the above.

Surgical Scar Revision

Surgical scar revision can be an effective solution for prominent or unsatisfactory scars. For optimal results it is highly advisable to have any surgical scar revision performed by a plastic surgeon.

➤ **When to Consider:** If you're dissatisfied with the appearance of your scars following non-surgical or topical scar treatments.

➤ **Ideal Candidates:** Individuals with <u>linear scars</u>, keloid scars, hypertrophic scars or scar contractures.

➤ **Procedure Overview:** Beyond excising and resuturing, Z-plasty and W-plasty may be done to reposition and reshape the existing scar tissue.

➤ **Risks:** Surgical revision of scars does carry risk of infection or that the new scar might not heal as expected, resulting in a scar that is not improved or could potentially look more noticeable.

➤ **Results:** Improvement to the scar will generally be noticeable within six to eight weeks, with long term stabilisation of the scar tissue and reduction in redness. Scar width and overall appearance can be properly assessed over six to 12 months.

Four Types of Non-Surgical Scar Treatments

Non surgical scar treatments may require several treatments spaced six weeks apart for the best results. Different treatments can also be combined and non-surgical treatments may also be utilised following scar revision surgery to further improve the appearance of scars.

Additionally, the success of non-surgical scar treatments depends on factors such as the qualifications of the practitioner, as well as the type and age of the scar, skin type, and your overall health. As with any medical intervention relating to cosmetic or plastic surgery, it's crucial to consult with a qualified plastic surgeon who can assess the specific characteristics of your scar and determine the most appropriate treatment plan for your individual case.

1. Steroid Injections

Steroid injections, specifically corticosteroids, are sometimes used as a treatment to reduce the thickness and improve the appearance of scars. Here's how they work:

➤ **Anti-inflammatory effects:** Corticosteroids have potent anti-inflammatory properties. Inflammation is a key factor in the development of hypertrophic and keloid scars. Injecting steroids directly into the scar tissue, can reduce inflammation, as well as redness, swelling, and itching associated with hypertrophic and keloid scars.

➤ **Inhibition of collagen production:** Hypertrophic and keloid scars are characterised by excessive collagen production. Collagen is a protein that plays a crucial role in wound healing, but an overproduction can lead to raised and thickened scars. Steroid injections help modulate collagen synthesis, preventing excessive buildup and promoting a more normalised healing response.

➤ **Softening and flattening of scars:** Steroid injections can lead to the softening and flattening of scars over time. This is particularly beneficial for hypertrophic and keloid scars, which tend to be raised and may cause discomfort or cosmetic concerns.

It's important to note that while steroid injections can be effective, multiple sessions may be required for optimal results.

Additionally, there are potential side effects associated with steroid injections, including skin atrophy (thinning of the skin), hypopigmentation (lightening of the skin), and the potential for the scar to become stretched and more noticeable when treatment commences..

2. Laser Therapy

Laser treatment for scars is a common and effective method used in dermatology and cosmetic surgery to reduce the appearance of scars. The process involves using laser light to target and break down scar tissue, stimulate collagen production, and encourage the growth of new, healthier skin cells.

Different types of lasers are available, each with its unique properties and applications for specific scar types. Multiple sessions may be required for optimal results, typically spaced six to eight weeks apart. Here's an overview of the laser treatment process and the various lasers used for scar treatment.

➤ **Fractional Laser:** Fractional lasers create micro-injuries in the skin, promoting collagen remodelling. Laser treatment is effective for reducing the appearance of various types of scars, including surgical scars.

➤ **Pulsed Dye Laser (PDL):** PDL targets blood vessels, reducing redness and promoting scar fading. This treatment is Ideal for reducing the appearance of red or vascular scars, such as hypertrophic scars and keloids.

➤ **CO_2 Laser:** CO_2 lasers remove layers of skin, stimulating collagen production and improving skin texture. Especially effective for treatment of deeper scars, especially atrophic surgical scars.

➤ **Nd:YAG Laser:** Nd:YAG lasers target blood vessels and pigmentation, reducing redness and discoloration. It can be used for the treatment of hypertrophic scars, keloids, and pigmented scars.

It's essential to note that the choice of laser depends on individual factors such as skin type, scar type, and the desired outcome. Consultation with a qualified plastic surgeon or dermatologist is crucial as lasers when used by an inexperienced practitioner can cause burns and make scars more noticeable. Always follow post-treatment care instructions to ensure a safe and effective recovery.

3. Intense Pulsed Light (IPL)

Intense Pulsed Light (IPL) targets melanin and haemoglobin, reducing discoloration and helping to even out skin tone. Treatment with IPL is normally recommended for scars with hyperpigmentation or redness.The visibility of the scar will determine how many treatments you need. It could take multiple treatments to improve some scars. IPL treatments can be carried out every four to eight weeks in order to get the desired effects.

4. Microneedling for Scar Treatment

The micro-injuries created during microneedling encourage the remodelling of scar tissue, leading to a smoother and more even skin surface. Microneedling is often performed as a series of sessions, spaced several weeks apart, to achieve optimal results.

While microneedling is generally considered safe for many people, it's essential to disclose your complete medical history, including any medications you are taking and consult with a qualified dermatologist to assess your individual case. You may not be suitable for microneedling if you have:

- Active skin infections or a chronic skin condition like eczema or psoriasis
- A history of forming keloid or hypertrophic scars
- Blood clotting disorders or require blood-thinning medications
- Undergone recent radiation therapy in the treatment area.

Topical Scar Treatment Options

Topical scar treatments can help the healing process, resulting in finer, flatter and more discreet scars. Products that have demonstrated an effect in clinical trials include:

➢ **Silicone scar products:** Available in the form of silicone sheets or silicone gel, silicone based products are commonly used in scar management to help scars heal and improve their appearance. The main mechanisms by which silicone scar treatments work is by improving hydration, making the scars more pliable.

This hydration has some effect on the inflammatory process helping to reduce hypertrophic and keloid scars.The semi-occlusive CICA-CARE Silicone Gel Sheet from Smith & Nephew is a medical-grade silicone sheet that helps hydrate the scar region and may lessen the thickness, itching, and colour of raised scars.

➢ **Scar creams and gels:** The majority of scar creams and gels have not been clinically proven to do anything more than nourish and hydrate skin. One scar cream that has been clinically shown to reduce the thickness and redness of scars is <u>Solution for Scars</u>. Importantly, it has also been shown that using the cream in advance of surgery gives significantly improved scar outcomes.

Conflict of Interest Declaration

The authors Annabelle Baugh and Mr Douglas McGeorge (FRCS) Plast report the following details of affiliation or involvement in the company Science of Skin (SOS), an organisation or entity with a financial interest in the subject matter or materials discussed in this section.

Final Thoughts

Choosing the right breast surgery scar treatment requires a combination of diligence and informed decision making. Whether opting for surgical or non-surgical interventions, or using topical solutions, consulting with your plastic surgeon will ensure a tailored approach to your unique needs.

Annabelle Baugh, Founder of Cosmetic Surgery Advancements

3. TRAVELLING ABROAD FOR COSMETIC SURGERY

TRAVELLING ABROAD FOR COSMETIC SURGERY

An increasing number of people are travelling abroad for cosmetic surgery procedures like breast augmentations, lifts or reductions. The appeal is clear - prices can be significantly cheaper even with travel costs factored in.

What Drives Lower Costs for Cosmetic Surgery Abroad?

Several key factors allow overseas clinics and hospitals to offer cosmetic surgery at significantly lower prices, these include:

➢ **Reduced labour costs** - The cost of cosmetic breast surgery is composed of professional, anaesthetic and hospital and consumable costs. Cosmetic surgeons, nurses and other medical staff earn considerably less in many countries compared to the UK, USA, Canada and Australia.

➢ **Exchange rates** - Weaker currencies in some countries can generate substantial savings after exchange rate conversions.

➢ **Lower Operational Overheads** - Lower real estate, administrative and maintenance costs overseas can mean that clinics and hospitals remain profitable while charging less.

➢ **Reduced Medication Expenses** - Breast implants and

other medical supplies tend to cost noticeably less in certain countries.

➢ **Standards** - Overseas hospitals may not be subjected to the same rigorous regulations that maintain high care standards in countries, such as the UK, USA, Canada and Australia.

Four Factors to Check for Cosmetic Breast Surgery Abroad

1. Your Plastic Surgeon

The most critical consideration is the actual surgeon you choose. Do extensive research to ensure your surgeon is fully qualified, licensed and credentialed in plastic surgery with the appropriate medical bodies.

There are various plastic surgery societies and associations as listed in Section One of this book. If you want to travel to a country that is not covered the other option is to find a plastic surgeon with membership to the International Society of Aesthetic Plastic Surgery (ISAPS).

The Benefits of Choosing an ISAPS Member Surgeon:

The ISAPS upholds rigorous selection criteria for their member surgeons. Approved candidates must meet high global benchmarks related to:

- **Certification** - Surgeons must be certified by legitimately-recognized bodies in their home countries to perform plastic surgery.
- **Years of training** - Extensive specialised training in aesthetic surgical procedures is required before consideration.

- **Procedure volume standards** - Surgeons must actively perform a high minimum number of cosmetic surgeries annually to demonstrate current experience.
- **Continuing education** - Ongoing participation in conferences and training programs is mandatory for remaining accredited.
- **Peer recommendations** - Fellow surgeons must vouch for a surgeon's quality of work, ethics and standards to qualify for ISAPS.

This thorough vetting process makes ISAPS membership a strong indicator of training and qualifications, safety practices and ethical integrity. Choosing an ISAPS-approved plastic surgeon provides confidence you have selected a recognised specialist for the best possible aesthetic outcome. No other international society upholds such rigorous membership criteria as a service to patients pursuing quality cosmetic surgery worldwide.

You should always have a consultation with the surgeon who will perform your procedure prior to making any payments. If this is done virtually you should also have an in person consultation prior to the procedure. Always check if you can get a refund if you decide not to go ahead and ask for the full terms and conditions in writing. READ THEM!

2. Breast Implants

If you are having breast surgery which involves a breast implant, request the breast implant manufacturer and the warranty details

3. Patient Reviews

Never rely on patient reviews or before and after photos from past patients as these can be fake or easily manipulated. Many cosmetic surgery companies will discourage patients from leaving negative reviews and will use legal action when a bad review is left on a third party review site.

4. The Medical Team and Facility

Along with credentials for the surgeon, the medical team should be properly qualified - ask for a list of the theatre support staff and nursing team and check each member of the team is registered with the appropriate medical bodies. Make sure the clinic or hospital meets standards for safety, cleanliness and has either an intensive care unit (ICU) or an arrangement in place with a hospital that can provide emergency care if required.

Medical Care and Cover

It is critical to discuss your medical care and cover beforehand with your overseas surgeon and medical facility. This includes:

➢ **Insurance provisions:** Personal travel insurance does not normally include cover for elective medical procedures abroad. Inquire what medical malpractice insurance and financial protections the surgeon and hospital have in place that specifically cover foreign patients. Also verify what costs will be covered if complications occur and you need to be transferred to another hospital.

➢ **Designated contacts:** Confirm who exactly you should contact in case of problems or unsatisfactory surgical results - get a specific point of contact on the medical team rather than a generic helpline. This should be a senior, English-speaking doctor fully capable of managing post-operative issues.

➢ **Discharge:** Check what the discharge criteria is for patients following this type of procedure and how you will be transported back to your hotel following the procedure.

➢ **Aftercare:** What happens if you need to be admitted into hospital for a complication after discharge and what type of medical cover is provided?

➤ **Revision surgery:** What revision surgery is provided and what medical cover and costs are covered in relation to complications or if you are not satisfied with the aesthetic outcome.

➤ **Accountability process:** Inquire as to the formal complaint or accountability process if you are dissatisfied with surgical outcomes or suffered complications. There should be a transparent, defined procedure for medical and financial responsibility.

Risks of Flying Post-Surgery

The NHS recommends waiting five to seven days as a minimum following breast surgery procedures. Staying in the country where your cosmetic breast surgery has been performed for at least 10 days and not returning until your stitches have dissolved (or are removed) and your incisions are healed is highly advisable. This allows for immediate follow-up care should any complications occur.

You also need to evaluate the risks of flying too soon after surgery. There is an increased risk for blood clots, swelling, pain and other complications. Discuss with your surgeon when it is safe to fly home, and plan your trip accordingly. Always wear support stockings on, both, outward and inward journeys.

Final Thoughts

Travelling abroad for cosmetic breast surgery may mean you can access a procedure that you can not afford in your country of residence. If you do decide to go abroad I would recommend choosing a country that you can easily return to for revision surgery if necessary.

There is no doubt that you can find qualified and experienced plastic surgeons and accredited medical facilities with high standards of care, in almost every country around the world. All surgery carries the risk of complications. Always do your own checks with external medical and regulatory bodies and have a plan for receiving care if complications arise once you return to your own country.

Annabelle Baugh, Founder of Cosmetic Surgery Advancements

4. ADVICE AND GUIDANCE

ADVICE AND GUIDANCE

Choosing to have cosmetic breast surgery is a deeply personal journey that requires a combination of self assurance, careful consideration, and effective communication. In this section, we provide tips on discussing your choices openly and compassionately with those who matter most and how to feel confident when making your final decision about your procedure.

Six Tips for Discussing Cosmetic Surgery with Friends and Family

1. Self-reflection and goal setting: Before diving into conversations with friends and family, take the time for self reflection. Identify your motivations and expectations for undergoing cosmetic breast surgery. Clearly define your goals to guide your decision-making process and your long term desired outcomes and communicate them effectively to others.

2. Researching surgeons and procedures: Choosing the right surgeon and surgical facility is crucial in ensuring a successful outcome. Research reputable plastic surgeons with expertise in the specific procedure you are considering. Being well informed about the surgical process will not only aid in your decision making but also help address concerns your friends and family may have.

3. Open and Honest Communication: Initiating open and honest communication with your friends and family is key to gaining their support. Choose an appropriate time and place to discuss your decision, emphasising your personal motivations and the research you have conducted. Be prepared to answer questions and address concerns they may have. Keep in mind that understanding and support may take time, so be patient and provide reassurance.

4. Share educational resources: To help your friends and family better understand the decision-making process, share educational resources about cosmetic breast surgery. Provide them with this book and links to reputable sites of plastic surgery organisations that explain the procedures, potential risks, and benefits. This information can help dispel myths and misconceptions, fostering a more informed and supportive environment.

5. Consider their perspectives: While your decision is ultimately yours to make, it's essential to consider the perspectives of your friends and family. Acknowledge their concerns and listen to their opinions with empathy. Addressing their worries and explaining your motivations may help alleviate their apprehensions and build a foundation of understanding.

6. Attend consultations together: If your loved ones are open to it, and you feel comfortable inviting concerned friends, partners or family to attend consultations with your chosen plastic surgeon can be extremely beneficial. This allows them to ask questions, gain insights into the procedure, and interact with medical professionals. Seeing the level of care and professionalism involved in the process can ease their concerns and provide additional reassurance.

Three Strategies for Confident Decision Making

1. Define your goals and motivations for undergoing cosmetic breast surgery.

2. Research different types of cosmetic breast surgery procedures to understand the various techniques and how they can impact the final results.

3. Create a comprehensive list of questions covering aspects such as the procedure details, techniques involved, and the specific ways in which the procedure aligns with your desired goals.

Guidelines for Selecting Your Plastic Surgeon

- Ensure the surgeon is certified by a recognised plastic surgery board, indicating specialised training and expertise in the field.
- Inquire about the number of years they have been practising and the frequency with which they perform the specific surgery.
- Verify that the procedure will be performed at an accredited hospital or surgical facility, ensuring adherence to safety standards.

Mastering the Consultation

➢ Discuss the techniques used to minimise risks and handle potential complications.

➢ Discuss the recovery time, potential risks, and long-term results associated with each procedure.

➢ Understand the impact of the surgery on future pregnancies or breastfeeding (if applicable).

➢ Get a detailed cost for the procedure and ensure it includes all potential post-operative expenses. Be careful not to use cost as your reasons for choosing a facility. Consider the whole package of care and who is providing it.

➤ Inquire about the post-operative care plan, including follow-up appointments, recovery guidelines, and availability for addressing any concerns.

Final Thoughts

By taking time to really think about the outcome you want to achieve and considering the risks and complications associated with the procedure you are considering you can make informed decisions about cosmetic breast surgery. Remember that your reasons and the feeling behind them are unique and not everyone will agree or understand why you want to have cosmetic breast surgery. Trust your inner feelings and if you still feel anxious about making a decision after a second consultation with your plastic surgeon, *consider seeking the help of a qualified counsellor or psychologist.*

Annabelle Baugh, Founder of Cosmetic Surgery Advancements.

5. FINAL THOUGHTS FROM ANNABELLE

1

FINAL THOUGHTS FROM ANNABELLE

Hello, my name is Annabelle and I'm the founder of Cosmetic Surgery Advancements (CSA). This book and organisation grew out of my personal experience with breast augmentation surgery. My final breast augmentation procedure was performed in 2002, I later learned that the breast implants I had chosen were recalled in 2019. This was due to their link to a rare immune system cancer called breast implant-associated anaplastic large cell lymphoma (BIA-ALCL).

At the time Allergan implants were widely considered among plastic surgeons to be one of the most trusted manufacturers of breast implants with an excellent safety record, so discovering this cancer risk scared and surprised me. My goal is that CSA will serve as a trustworthy resource, providing the latest research on risks like BIA-ALCL and information to help others make fully informed decisions when considering cosmetic surgery.

Reflecting on my own experience, I initially selected Mr Douglas McGeorge FRCS (Plast) based on a friend's recommendation. I was fortunate that he was not only a fully qualified plastic surgeon, but also extremely caring and always responded to my questions or concerns promptly.

Realising that my story could have taken a different turn if I had selected a surgeon based on testimonials or ratings, I became acutely aware that presently, global regulatory bodies are falling short in safeguarding patients' interests from unscrupulous 'cosmetic surgery' surgeons and organisations will prioritise profits over patients wellbeing and safety. It's this alarming scenario that prompted the creation of CSA's Cosmetic Surgery Directory, which strives to provide the highest calibre of plastic surgeons, in an industry that demands increased scrutiny.

Choosing a surgeon is such a personal decision. I want everyone considering cosmetic procedures to feel supported as your most authentic self—not reliant on promotions, testimonials or star ratings that don't tell the full story. I encourage you strongly to scrutinise qualifications thoroughly rather than going on potentially misleading recommendations alone.

My goal is that the Cosmetic Surgery Advancements website is always here to answer questions and back you up along the way with information that makes you feel confident and comfortable as you explore cosmetic surgery options. This should be an empowering process centred around self love. Please reach out through my site contact form for personalised guidance.

Be Your Most Authentic Self xxx
Annabelle Baugh, Founder of Cosmetic Surgery Advancements

RESEARCH AND RESOURCES

Maaløe R, Hansen CL, Pedersen T. Anaestesidødsfald. Definition, årsager, risikofaktorer og forebyggelse [Death under anesthesia. Definition, causes, risk factors and prevention]. Ugeskr Laeger. 1995 Nov 20;157(47):6561-5. From: PubMed

Cherobin ACFP, Tavares GT. Safety of local anesthetics. An Bras Dermatol. 2020 Jan-Feb;95(1):82-90. From: NCBI

Institute of Medicine (US) Committee on the Safety of Silicone Breast Implants; Bondurant S, Ernster V, Herdman R, editors. Safety of Silicone Breast Implants. Washington (DC): National Academies Press (US); 1999. 3, Implant Catalogue. From: NCBI

Fardo D, Sequeira Campos M, Pensler JM.. Breast Augmentation Last update 2023 July 18. From: NCBI

Patel BC, Wong CS, Wright T, et al. Breast Implants Updated 2022 Aug 1. From: NCBI

Daniel J Gould, Orr Shauly, Levonti Ohanissian, W Grant Stevens, Subfascial Breast Augmentation: A Systematic Review and Meta-Analysis of Capsular Contracture, Aesthetic Surgery Journal Open Forum, Volume 2, Issue 1, January 2020. From: ASJOF

Jeffrey M. Jacobson, Margaret E. Gatti, Adam D. Schaffner, Lauren M. Hill, Scott L. Spear, Effect of Incision Choice on Outcomes in Primary Breast Augmentation, Aesthetic Surgery Journal, Volume 32, Issue 4, May 2012, Pages 456–462, From: ASJ

FDA warns of risks from breast implants From: PMC

UPDATE: Reports of Squamous Cell Carcinoma (SCC) in the Capsule Around Breast Implants. From: FDA Safety Communication

Breast Augmentation: A Risk Factor for Breast Cancer? June 18, 1992 N Engl J Med 1992; 326:1649-1653 From: NEJMJenny Carvajal, Jairo H. Patiña, Mammographic Findings After Breast Augmentation With Autologous Fat Injection, Aesthetic Surgery Journal, Volume 28, Issue 2, March 2008, Pages 153–162. From: Aesthetic Surgery Journal

Ørholt, Mathias B.M.Sc.; Larsen, Andreas B.M.Sc.; Hemmingsen, Mathilde N. B.M.Sc.; Mirian, Christian M.D.; Zocchi, Michele L. M.D., Ph.D.; Vester-Glowinski, Peter V. M.D., Ph.D.; Herly, Mikkel M.D. Complications after Breast Augmentation with Fat Grafting: A Systematic Review. Plastic and Reconstructive Surgery 145(3):p 530e-537e, March 2020.From: Plastic and Reconstructive Surgery Journal

Preliminary Opinion on the safety of breast implants in relation to anaplastic large cell lymphoma 20201116. Presented by Wim H. De Jong, DVM, PhD. Scientific Committee on Health, Environment and Emerging Risks (SCHEER) DG Health and Food Safety European Commission.

Breast Implants: Reports of Squamous Cell Carcinoma and Various Lymphomas in Capsule Around Implant. From: FDA Safety Communication

UPDATE: Reports of Squamous Cell Carcinoma (SCC) in the Capsule Around Breast Implants. From: FDA Safety Communication

Breast Implant Associated Anaplastic Large Cell Lymphoma (BIA-ALCL) Information for patients, public and health care professionals. MHRA 26 July 2017 Last updated 28 April 2023. From: GOV.UK Guidance

Breast implants and anaplastic large cell lymphoma. Update - Suspended breast implant devices now cancelled Published 29 October 2020, Last updated 7 February 2023 From: TGA

Lynch EB, DeCoster RC, Vyas KS, Rinker BD, Yang M, Vasconez HC, Clemens MW. Current risk of breast implant-associated anaplastic large cell lymphoma: a systematic review of epidemiological studies. Vol 5 30 September 2021. From: ABS Annals of Breast Surgery

Tevis SE, Hunt KK, Clemens MW. Stepwise En Bloc Resection of Breast Implant-Associated Anaplastic Large Cell Lymphoma with Oncologic Considerations. Aesthet Surg J Open Forum. 2019 Feb 27. From: PubMed

Institute of Medicine (US) Committee on the Safety of Silicone Breast Implants; Bondurant S, Ernster V, Herdman R, editors. Safety of Silicone Breast Implants. Washington (DC): National Academies Press (US); 1999. 9, Silicone Breast Implants and Cancer. From: NCBI

Salzman MJ. Silent Rupture of Silicone Gel Breast Implants: High-Resolution Ultrasound Scans and Surveys of 584 Women. Plast Reconstr Surg. 2022 Jan 1;149(1):7-14.From: PRS

Ann Surg Treat Res. 2017 Dec;93(6):331-335. English.
Published online Dec 01, 2017. From: ASTR

Hillard C, Fowler JD, Barta R, Cunningham B. Silicone breast implant rupture: a review. Gland Surg. 2017 Apr;6(2):163-168. From: PMCID: PMC

European Journal of Radiology, Volume 53, Issue 2, February 2005, Pages 213-225
The diagnosis of breast implant rupture: MRI findings compared with findings at explantation

Lisbet R. Hölmich, Ilse Vejborg, Carsten Conrad, Susanne Sletting, Joseph K. McLaughlin From: ScienceDirect

What is capsular contracture and how can it be treated? From: ASPS

Zhang, Z., Qi, J., Zhang, X. et al. What Can We Learn from Breast Implant Explantation: a 28-Year, Multicenter Retrospective Study of 1004 Explantation Cases. Aesth Plast Surg 47, 1743–1750 (2023). From: Springer

Medor MC, Bouhadana G, Churchill IF, Hemmerling T, Bonapace-Potvin M,

Papanastasiou C, Mussie A, Borsuk DE, Papanastasiou VW. How Big Is Too Big? Exploring the Relationship between Breast Implant Volume and Postoperative Complication Rates in Primary Breast Augmentations. Plast Reconstr Surg Glob Open. 2023 Mar 8;11(3):e4843. From: PRS

Swanson, Eric MD. Underestimating Implant Volumes in Cosmetic Breast Augmentation. Plastic and Reconstructive Surgery - Global Open 5(9):p e1483, September 2017. From: PRS

Ramanadham, Smita R. MD, FACS*; Rose Johnson, Anna MD, MPH†. Breast Lift with and without Implant: A Synopsis and Primer for the Plastic Surgeon. Plastic and Reconstructive Surgery - Global Open 8(10):p e3057, October 2020. From: PRS

Breast Reduction Techniques and Outcomes: A Meta-analysis
Stephen P. Daane, MD, W. Bradford Rockwell, MD
Aesthetic Surgery Journal, Volume 19, Issue 4, July 1999, Pages 293–303, From: ASJ

Current surgical techniques for nipple reduction: A literature review
Hannah Trøstrup, Iselin Saltvig, Steen Henrik Matzen
Open Access, July 17. From: JPRAS

Nagaraja Rao D, Winters R. Inverted Nipple. [Updated 2023 July 4]. From: NCBI

Update on the Treatment of Scars, Volume 18, Issue 6, June 2019. From: JDD

www.ingramcontent.com/pod-product-compliance
Lightning Source LLC
Chambersburg PA
CBHW052201220526
45471CB00004B/1769